IMAGES
of America

TRAVERSE CITY
STATE HOSPITAL

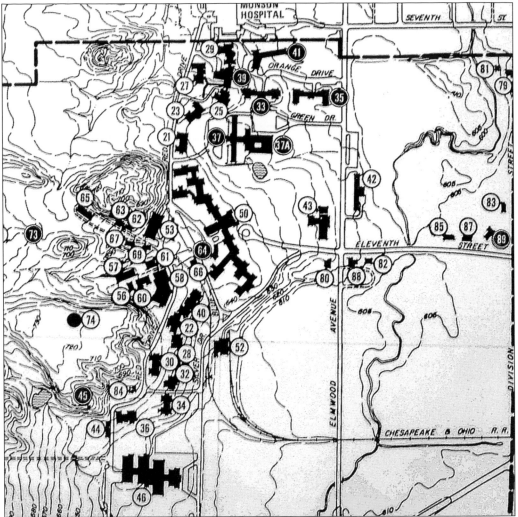

MAP OF TRAVERSE CITY STATE HOSPITAL, 1970S. This map reflects the grounds and buildings as Traverse City State Hospital stood in the 1970s. The only alteration to the original map is that buildings now demolished or removed (such as 41, 89, and others) are designated with white letters in a black circle. Some of the grounds are off the edge, such as the farm buildings to the south. None of the newer construction and alterations, such as Grand Traverse Pavilions and Medical Campus Drive, are reflected on this map.

IMAGES
of America

TRAVERSE CITY
STATE HOSPITAL

Chris Miller

ARCADIA
PUBLISHING

Published by Arcadia Publishing
Charleston, South Carolina

Printed in the United States of America

Library of Congress Catalog Card Number: 2004117610

For all general information contact Arcadia Publishing at:
Telephone 843-853-2070
Fax 843-853-0044
E-mail sales@arcadiapublishing.com
For customer service and orders:
Toll-Free 1-888-313-2665

Visit us on the Internet at www.arcadiapublishing.com

*I dedicate this book to my sons, Jack and Benjamin Miller, and also
to the patients and staff of Traverse City State Hospital.*

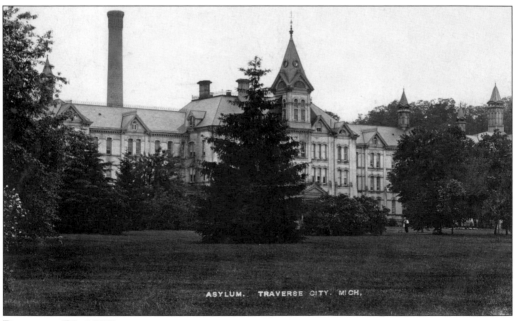

BUILDING 50, 1907.

CONTENTS

ACKNOWLEDGMENTS

This book was made possible by the efforts of many who have worked to preserve the history of Traverse City Hospital. Special thanks for their help with this project are due to: Heidi Johnson, Brian Upton, Julius Petertyl, Paul Hansen, Lois Orth, Donna Miller, Phil Balyeat, Bob Wilhelm, Ray Minervini, Raymond Minervini II, Steve Harold, Bob Wilson, Dan Truckey, Gary Curtiss, Dr. Jerry Linenger, Jerry Konczal, Joan Julin, Jim Anderson, Tracy Kurtz, Fred Lortet, Mike Long, Eric Erickson, C.S. Wright, Mark Stone, Anne Hoopfer, Dee Talantis, George Beckett, Louis Bass, Ken Christensen, Grand Traverse Pavilions, Adrienne Hoxie, the Minervini Group, Larry Wakefield, Janet Hibbard, Gene Hibbard, Members Credit Union, Wayne Moody, Ken Richmond, the Con Foster Museum, Gary Miller, Joyce Walter, Robert Bogdan, Robert Foster, Mike Long, Bradley Upham, Lew Razek, Ed Barty, the Archives of the State of Michigan, the Grand Traverse Pioneer and Historical Society, and the firm of Wigen, Tincknell, Meyer and Associates.

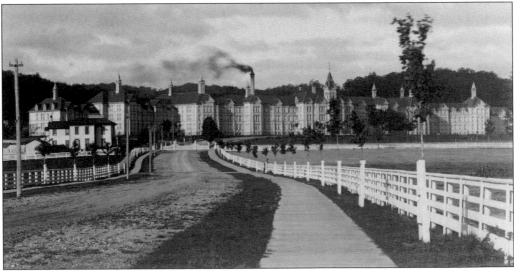

NORTHERN MICHIGAN ASYLUM, 1900. (Courtesy of Wayne Moody.)

INTRODUCTION

During the last half of the 19th century, many states began building large institutions to care for their citizens who had mental illnesses. The recommendations of Dr. Thomas Story Kirkbride dominated the design of these asylums. This plan included large imposing symmetric asylum buildings with ventilation towers and many other specifications relating to architecture and management. Many psychiatric hospitals designed on the "Kirkbride plan" were constructed throughout the nation. The first one in Michigan was in Kalamazoo, followed by a second one in Pontiac. These hospitals quickly filled up, and the State of Michigan found a need for another.

Looking to the future when the lumber would run out and the city would need another industry to thrive, Perry Hannah ("the father of Traverse City") used his influence with the state to secure Traverse City as the location for the new Northern Michigan Asylum. Opened in 1885, the institution remained one of the area's major employers (and a significant part of the local economy) until its closing. The first building opened was a massive Kirkbride-plan structure known today as Building 50.

Under the guidance of the first superintendent, Dr. James Decker Munson, the institution grew, and within just a few years of Building 50's opening, new buildings were added to handle a growing patient population. This included "cottage" housing for patients, which became popular as the Kirkbride plan fell out of favor. Dr. Munson believed that "beauty is therapy," and he strove to make the grounds beautiful. He also believed that "work is therapy," providing patients opportunities to work on the farms and in other positions necessary to keep the institution self-sufficient.

During the 1930s, large college-like buildings were constructed on the northwest side of the grounds, representing another shift in philosophies of psychiatric care. By the late 1970s, the main asylum building wings constructed in 1885 were completely abandoned, with patient activities mostly taking place in the 1930s buildings and in newer buildings. These buildings are very important in the community memory, as there are many people in Traverse City today who worked in them or used their services.

Early on, Dr. Munson was driven to serve the medical needs of Traverse City's citizens as well, and he started a general hospital in one of the State Hospital buildings in 1915. Later, shortly after Munson's death, a new brick medical hospital was constructed in the northern part of the state hospital grounds, and this hospital was operated by the state until the 1950s, when it became a separate entity. Now rivaling the old psychiatric hospital in building space, Munson

Medical Center is Traverse City's largest employer, and is equipped to provide critical care to patients from a surrounding 22-county area.

Changes in budget priorities, new laws (such as the one which closed the farm operation), changes in mental health care philosophy, and the introduction of new medications for treatment combined to cause the decline of the institution from the 1950s until its closure in 1989.

In 1980, the State of Michigan attempted to demolish four of the south cottages, but this destruction was halted by City Commissioner Carol Hale and others in the community. It was the first of many struggles in modern times to preserve the historic buildings and lands from demolition and other threats. After Traverse City State Hospital closed, the area was renamed Grand Traverse Commons. The community struggled throughout the 1990s with how to preserve, re-use, and restore the historic and natural resources of this large area. Some of the less-historic large buildings from the 1930s and later were demolished to make way for construction related to medical care and senior housing needed by the community. After the turn of the 21st century, however, everything else began to fall into place for the future preservation of the grounds and historic buildings.

Far from being a shuttered-away complex of abandoned buildings, the former State Hospital area has come to be known as "Traverse City's Central Park." The highly accessible grounds and trails are used for recreation, and the buildings are put to new uses. It also has become a hub of business activity as more and more offices open up in Building 50. Photographers and artists frequently visit the grounds to paint, sketch, and photograph the features.

Now owned by the Minervini Group, Building 50 (still the centerpiece) is well o the way to completely renovation into a mixed-use community of residences, offices, restaurants, and shops. A non-profit group, Rolling Centuries Farm, is making progress in preserving and rehabilitating the historic barns left over from the farming operation. Several of the cottages have been fully rehabilitated, and it is certain that the rest will be restored also. Other buildings, ranging from the oldest building (a farmhouse that dates back to 1879) to the much more recent All Faiths Chapel, have also found new uses.

This book contains photographs, maps, and other images that reflect the history of what started out as Northern Michigan Asylum, became Traverse City State Hospital (the name remembered by most), closed under the name of Traverse City Regional Psychiatric Hospital, and is now known as Grand Traverse Commons.

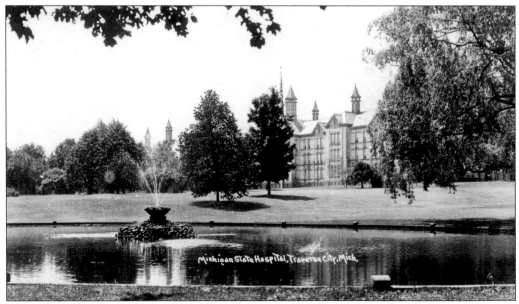

BUILDING 50 AND POND, 1960s.

One

BEGINNINGS

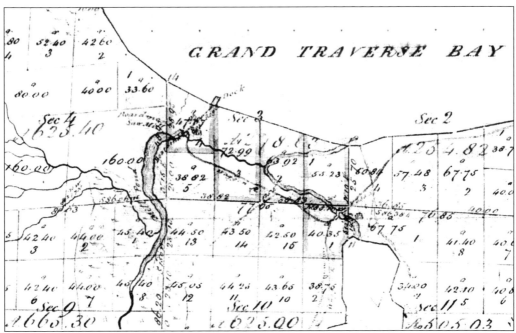

SURVEY MAP. This survey map is from 1851, more than 30 years before Northern Michigan Asylum was founded. The wide body of water running north to south was the mill pond for Horace Boardman's sawmill, which was located near what is now the corner of 3rd Street and Division (the northeast end of the long pond on the map). The future state hospital grounds are in the lower left area, to the southwest of the mill pond. In the early years of Traverse City's history, lumber was most important. (Courtesy of the Grand Traverse Pioneer and Historical Society.)

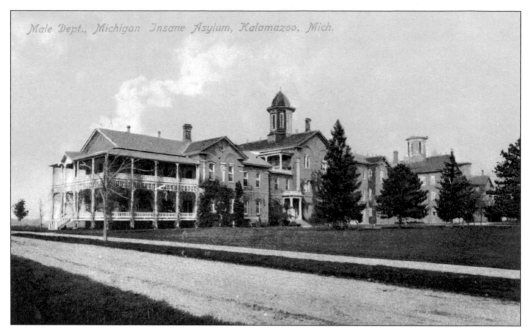

Male Dept., Michigan Insane Asylum, Kalamazoo, Mich.

POSTCARD VIEW OF ASYLUM AT KALAMAZOO, 1909. Inspired by the urgings of reformers such as Dorothea Dix, and the ideas of Dr. Thomas Story Kirkbride of Pennsylvania Hospital in Philadelphia, Michigan built its first "Kirkbride plan" psychiatric hospital in Kalamazoo in 1858. The first superintendent was Edwin H. Van Deusen.

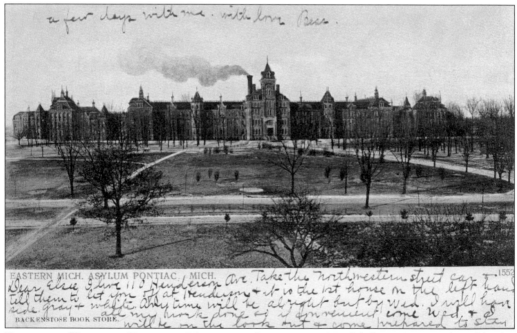

POSTCARD VIEW OF EASTERN MICHIGAN ASYLUM, 1907. Michigan's second Kirkbride-inspired psychiatric institution was built in Pontiac, Michigan, in 1878. For many of its early years, Dr. Henry M. Hurd was the superintendent. Shortly after it was completed, the State of Michigan found that there was a need to expand psychiatric services with a third hospital.

PERRY HANNAH. Perry Hannah, known to this day as "the Father of Traverse City," worked hard to get Michigan's next asylum located in Traverse City. He knew that the lumber would give out eventually, and that Traverse City needed another major source of employment to keep its economy going in future years.

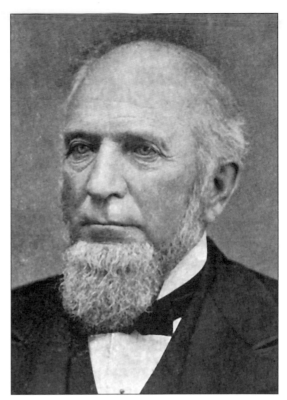

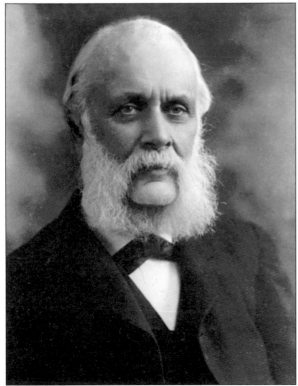

GORDON W. LLOYD. Gordon W. Lloyd (1832–1904), the architect contracted to design Northern Michigan Asylum, was one of the Midwest's foremost church architects. Born in England, he trained at England's Royal Academy. He immigrated to the United States in 1858 and settled in the Detroit area. Aside from many churches in Michigan, Ohio, and elsewhere, he also designed Grace Hospital in Detroit and Dowling Hall of the University of Detroit. (From the Jack Kausch Collection.)

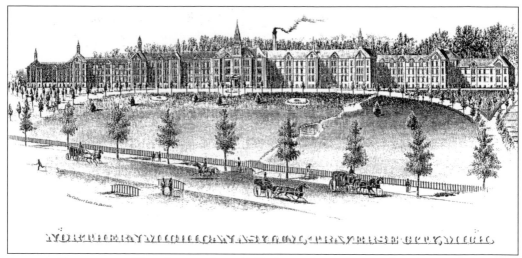

ASYLUM RENDERING. This drawing from 1882 shows the asylum as the planners envisioned it before its construction. In this rendition, the wings all recede from the center at 90-degree angles (in typical Kirkbride fashion). Building 50 was constructed with some variance in these angles in order to better fit the site and to provide better views of West Grand Traverse Bay.

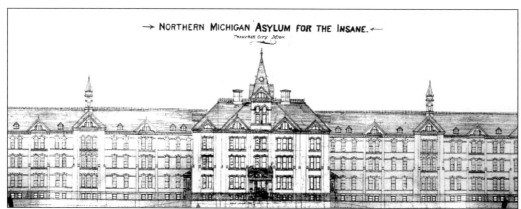

ARCHITECT'S RENDERING OF BUILDING 50. This architect's drawing depicts plans for the front elevation of Building 50. Old Center and the center sections are shown. The northern and southern ends of the building go beyond the edge of this image. In 1882, Gordon W. Lloyd said of his design, "The building front is of Italian character. Modified by considerations of expense and climate, avoiding elaborate detail . . . a general aspect of suitability to its purpose and an avoidance of all purely decorative features." (Courtesy of the State Archives of Michigan.)

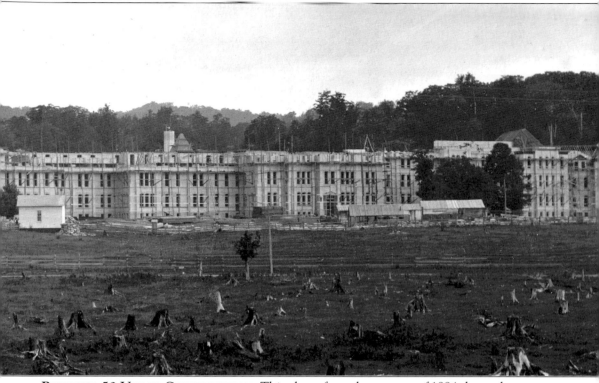

BUILDING 50 UNDER CONSTRUCTION. This photo from the summer of 1884 shows the center sections of Building 50 under construction. The dark main entrance in Old Center can be seen in the middle of the photograph. The stumps seen in the foreground would later be removed to create the "great lawn." (Courtesy of the Con Foster Museum.)

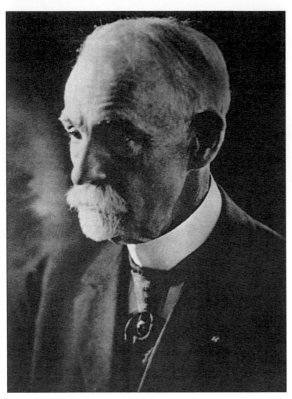

DR. JAMES DECKER MUNSON. James Decker Munson was brought in to be the first acting superintendent of the asylum just before it opened in November of 1885. He served from September 3, 1885, to July 1, 1924. A painting version of this photograph hangs in the lobby of Munson Medical Center. (Courtesy of the Grand Traverse Pioneer and Historical Society.)

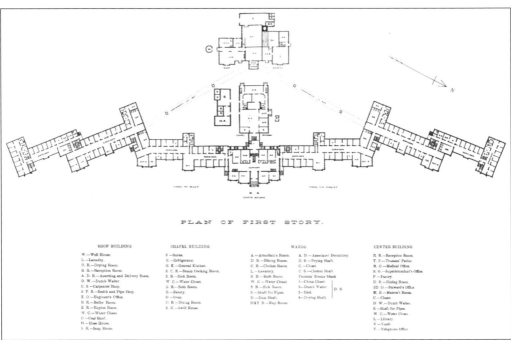

ASYLUM FLOOR PLAN. This floor plan shows the layout of the asylum in its first decade. This layout is typical of other Kirkbride-plan asylums: administration in the center, patient wings on either side, and a chapel and other functions to the rear of the center.

Two

BUILDING 50

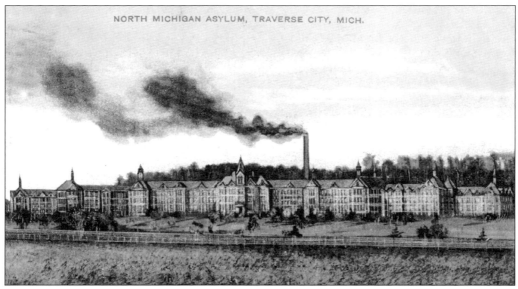

NORTH MICHIGAN ASYLUM, TRAVERSE CITY, MICH.

BUILDING 50, 1909. This postcard, mailed in 1909, shows the eastern elevation of the entire Northern Michigan Asylum main building. This building is now known as Building 50. The extreme left and right ends in this view are two-story wings, which would be changed into three-story wings by 1910. The southern (left) half of the building was for male patients, and the northern (right) half was for females. For most of the history of the institution, Building 50 was the hub of activity, and it remains the largest and most architecturally significant building of the complex.

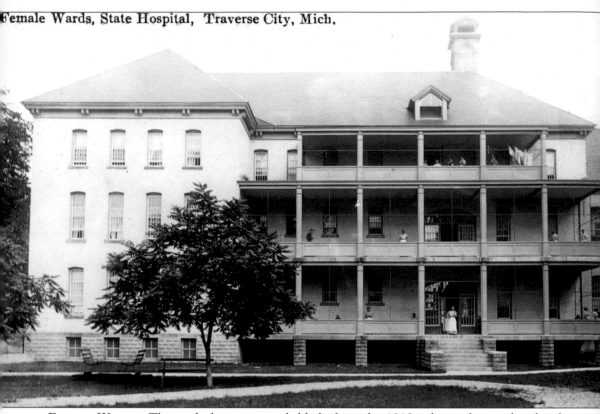

FEMALE WARDS. This real photo postcard, likely from the 1910s, shows the south side of the very north end of Building 50. This is the section where the most severely affected female patients resided. The first floor is Hall 5, the second floor is Hall 11, and the third floor is Hall 17. The main reasons for admission to the asylum (from an 1892 list) included puerperal (after childbirth), epilepsy, ill health, and intemperance. Some of the more obscure reasons for patient admission included business reversal, religious excitement, seduction, and nostalgia. (Courtesy of Heidi Johnson.)

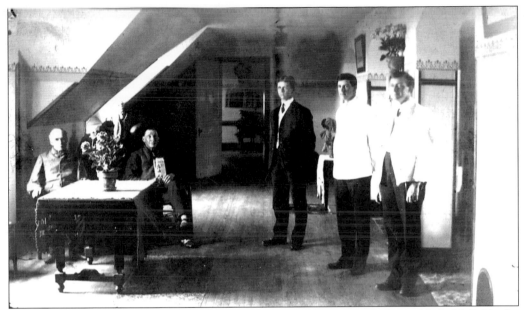

HALL 18. This very old photograph shows men in the attic area of what is likely Hall 18, the uppermost floor of the southernmost wing of Building 50. (Courtesy of Julius Petertyl.)

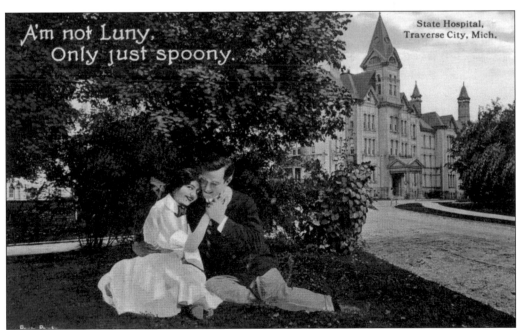

"LUNY SPOONY" POSTCARD, 1914. This postcard was one of a large number of postcards created by Orson W. Peck. Peck mailed this particular one to his son in 1914. He wrote on the back: "One of my new ones that just came in. Did you ever have the Luny Spoony feeling? This card ought to make quite a bit, don't you think? O.W.P." (Courtesy of George Beckett.)

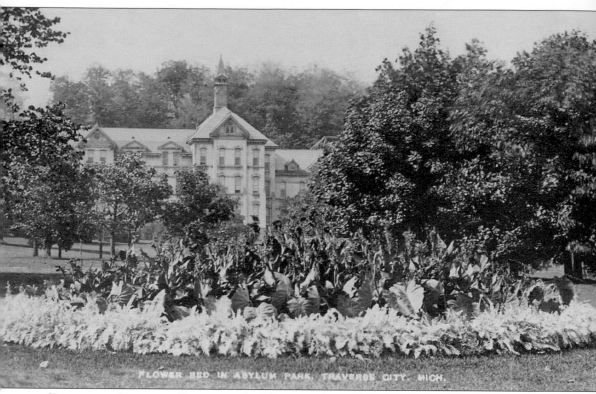

FLOWER BED IN ASYLUM PARK, TRAVERSE CITY, MICH.

FLOWERS IN FRONT OF BUILDING 50. This view shows the eastern elevation of the middle of the northern (women's) wing of Building 50. This particular version is from a real photo postcard mailed in 1909. There were several different editions of this postcard printed, each with subtle differences in coloration and lettering. The flowers in the foreground are dusty miller encircling canna. This type of planting was popular in Victorian times, and was found elsewhere on the state hospital grounds. A park bench dedicated to former grounds superintendant Earle Steele (1914–2003) is now found in the area seen in this view.

18

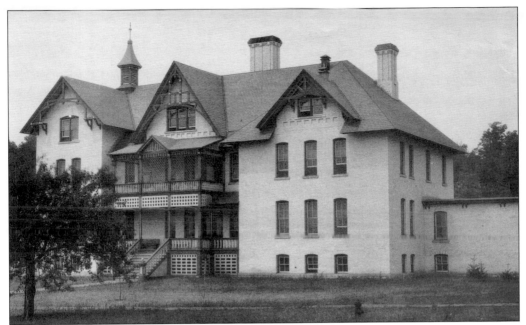

HALL 20 (INFIRMARY), C. 1900. This is an image of the southern elevation of the Infirmary for Males. After its construction, it was attached to the back end of Building 50 by a one-story hall (seen to the right). This infirmary, like the identical one attached to the women's wing of Building 50, was completed by 1890 in order to meet the medical needs of the patients. (Courtesy of Heidi Johnson.)

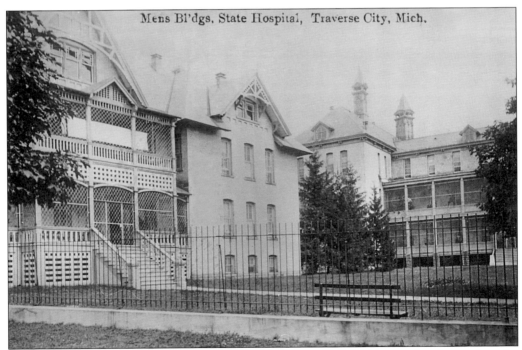

HALL 20 COURTYARD. This vintage postcard view shows Hall 20 (the men's infirmary) to the left, with the rear of the men's wing of Building 50 to the right. (Courtesy of Heidi Johnson.)

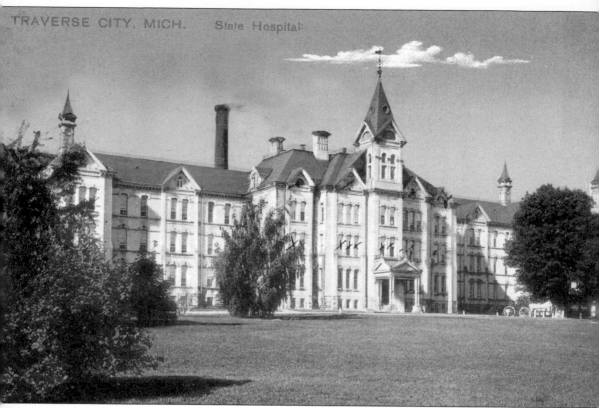

LIVING IN OLD CENTER, 1913. This Orson W. Peck postcard mailed from Traverse City in 1913 bears the message: "Got back O.K. How do you like my home. The crosses on top is where I work. Friend, S.E.H." The crosses referred to are X's in the windows of the center section above the entrance. (Courtesy of George Beckett.)

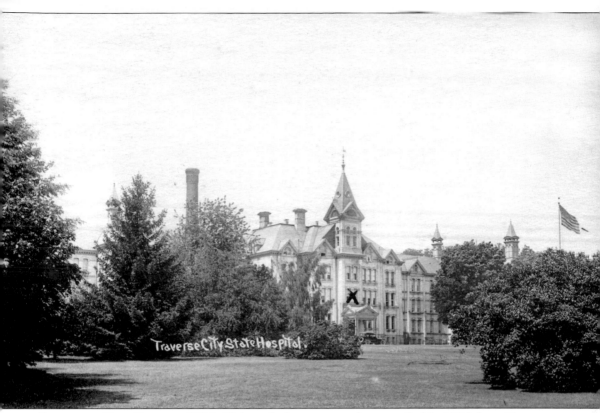

LIVING IN OLD CENTER, 1926. This real photo postcard was mailed in 1926 from Traverse City to Kalamazoo. Written on the back is the message: "Dear Brownie, I wish you could have been here to hear the address by Bishop Fisher which he gave this morning. It was wonderful. The cross on the picture indicates our room. It sure is a wonderful place. Goodby Brownie. Sid." The cross is above the entrance. (Courtesy of George Beckett.)

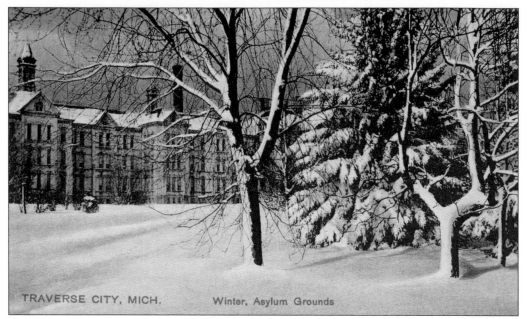

TRAVERSE CITY, MICH.   Winter, Asylum Grounds

BUILDING 50 IN WINTER, C. 1910. This c. 1910 postcard shows the front of the southern half of Building 50 during winter. This view is much the same now, except that the smokestack in the background is gone and the trees are different.

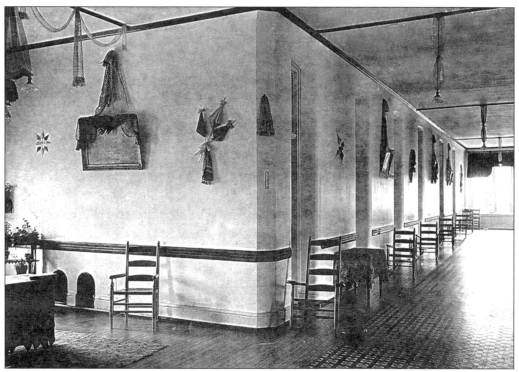

HALL 5. This photo from the early years of the institution shows Hall 5, which is the first floor of the north end of Building 50. Halls 11 and 17 are above it. (Courtesy of the State Archives of Michigan.)

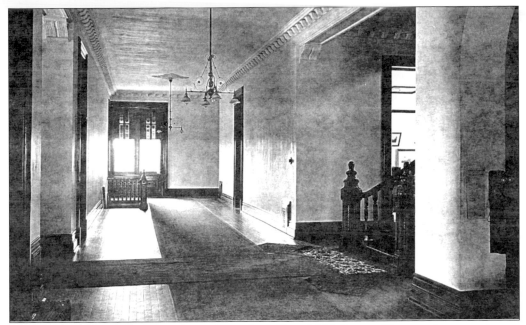

LOBBY OF OLD CENTER. This photo shows the lobby of Old Center. The grand open staircase, seen on the right, is listed as the main reason for the demolition of Old Center because it was a fire hazard. (Courtesy of the State Archives of Michigan.)

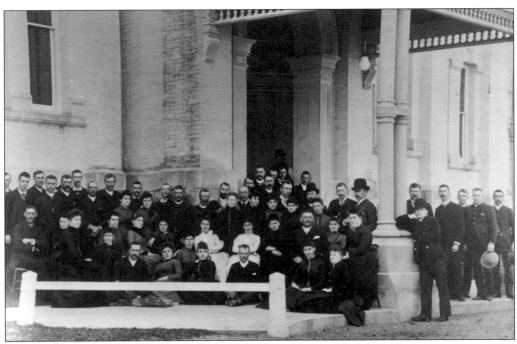

MAIN ENTRANCE. A group of male and female state hospital employees pose in front of the ornate pillars of Old Center's main entrance in this photo from the institution's early years. Photographs of actual patients at the state hospital are rare because of restrictions to protect confidentiality. (Courtesy of the State Archives of Michigan.)

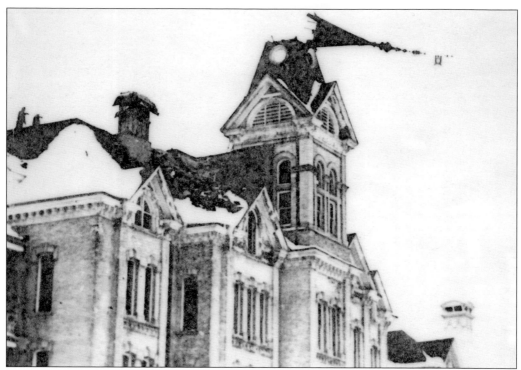

DEMOLITION OF OLD CENTER BEGINS. This photo shows Old Center at the start of demolition on January 8, 1963. Two men can be seen standing on the roof to the left. The top of the spire is bent to a 90-degree angle. (Courtesy of the State Archives of Michigan.)

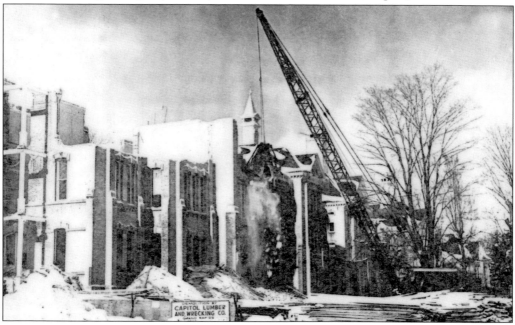

DEMOLITION OF OLD CENTER CONTINUES. The demolition of Old Center by Capitol Wrecking and Lumber Company of Grand Rapids, Michigan, continues in this photograph. (Courtesy of the State Archives of Michigan.)

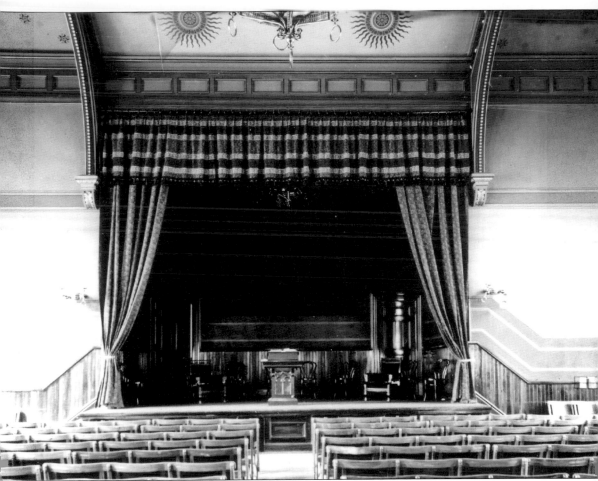

ALTAR AREA OF CHAPEL. The chapel section located to the west of the center of Building 50 was part of Gordon W. Lloyd's original design. However, the service buildings that were originally to the west of it no longer remain, and it now connects to Building 50's new center section instead of the original center. The chapel was last used as a library, and nothing remains of the ornate decoration seen here except for some of the woodwork near the ceiling. (Courtesy of the State Archives of Michigan.)

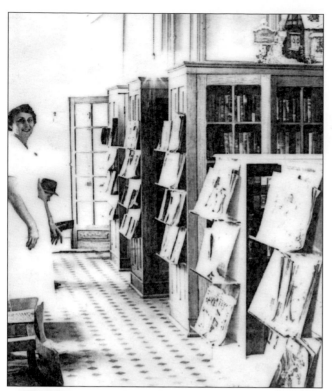

PATIENT LIBRARY. In the 1930s, the chapel was converted into a patient library. Chapel functions were moved elsewhere (such as the women's auditorium, and later the All Faith s Chapel). The bookshelves remained in the room until the late 1990s. (Courtesy of the State Archives of Michigan.)

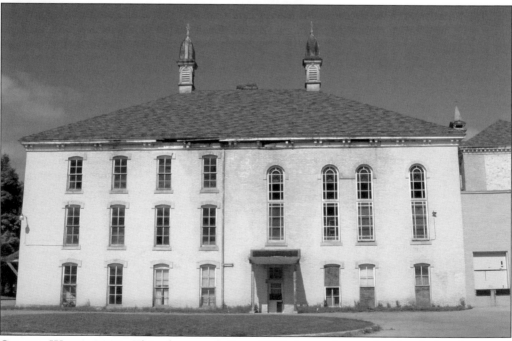

CHAPEL WING, 2003. This photograph from 2003 shows the south side of chapel wing of Building 50. The arched windows to the right have colored glass around the edges. The rusty spires seen on this photo were painted in 2004 and now have red tops. This section was constructed in 1885 as part of Building 50.

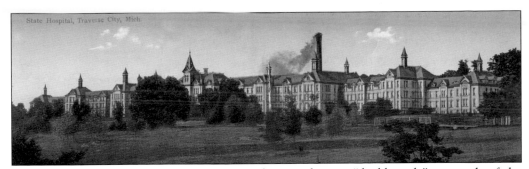

POSTCARD FROM MRS. MUNSON. Orsen Peck printed many "double-wide" postcards of the Grand Traverse region, including a few of the state hospital. This particular bears a message from Dr. Munson's wife, Marion Munson, reading, "Traverse City, May 29, 1913. My Dear Mr. and Mrs. Whitney, We reached home May Third. The weather has been cold all through this month. Doctor has not been well, had two bad spells, and has suffered much, has great difficulty in breathing. Today is a bit the warmer, and he feels better. I have wished many times that we were back in S.F. We enjoyed a visit from Bishop McCormick last Sunday. I feer we did not express our appreciation of all your mindless to us in Calif. When you come to Mich. we hope to have the pleasure of entertaining you. You will pardon my delay in letting you know of our safe arrival. I have led a strenuous life since I got home. With kind regards from us both, to both of you. Marion Munson." John J. McCormick was the Episcopalian bishop for the West Michigan region from 1909 to 1937.

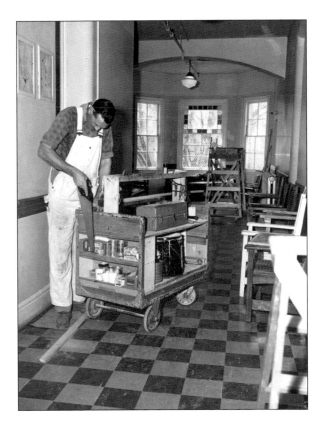

MAINTENANCE WORK.
Maintenance worker Bob Slater is shown here working in either Hall 19 or Hall 20 in the early 1970s. The Minervini Group is carefully preserving interesting features of the buildings, including the colored glass in the window frames found in the westward-facing bay windows of Hall 19 and Hall 20. (Courtesy of Paul Hansen.)

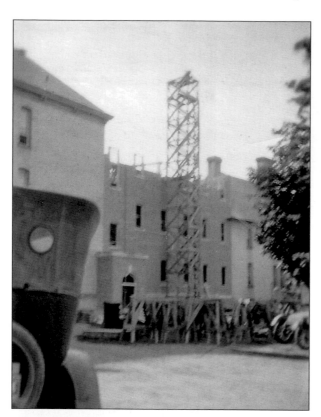

FRY WING UNDER CONSTRUCTION, 1930S. The "Fry Wing" is shown here under construction. It replaced an earlier one-story wing that connected the rear of Building 50 to Hall 20. It was designed by Lynn W. Fry of the State Building Departmentand used as nurses' dormitories. Fry also designed buildings at the Michigan State Fairgrounds. (Courtesy of Julius Petertyl.)

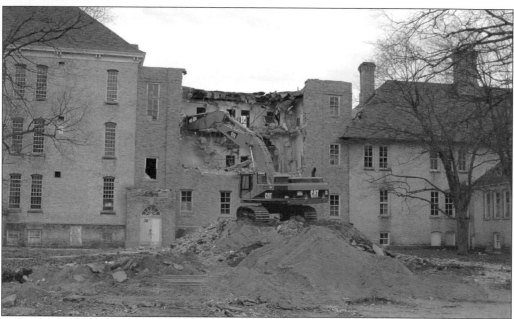

FRY WING BEING DEMOLISHED, 2003. During November of 2003, the Fry Wing connecting Building 50 with Hall 20 was demolished. At the time, this was the only section of Building 50 that was to be demolished. This wing had been severely damaged due to deterioration that occurred after the building closed.

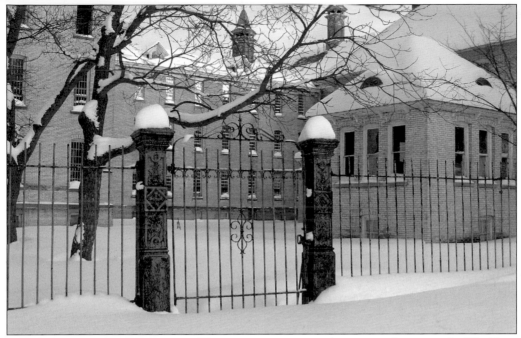

NORTH COURTYARD GATE, 2004. The ornate iron gate at the rear north courtyard of Building 50 is a beautiful spot favored by photographers and artists.

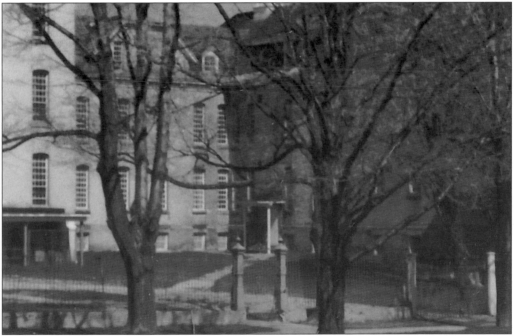

SOUTH COURTYARD GATE, 1980. This photograph from 1980 shows the gate and fence at the south courtyard (south of Hall 20). Long since removed, the gate was very similar to the one that still remains at the north courtyard. The area behind the gate is now one of the entrances to Trattoria Stella. (Courtesy of Julius Petertyl.)

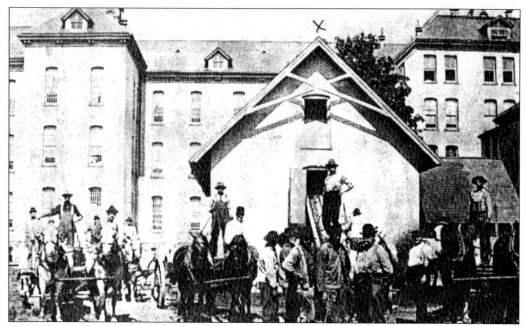

MEAT MARKET. The meat market behind Building 50 is shown in this photograph from the 1910s or 1920s. The men are filling a cooler with ice. Robert Herkner was the head meat cutter. Located to the north of the chapel, this building was demolished in the 1940s. (Courtesy of Julius Petertyl.)

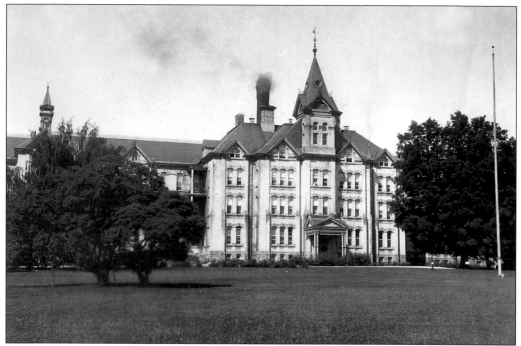

GREAT LAWN. This photo, c. 1925, looks across the "great lawn" toward the Old Center of Building 50. This open lawn remains today as one of the cherished natural features of the Grand Traverse Commons property. (Courtesy of Julius Petertyl.)

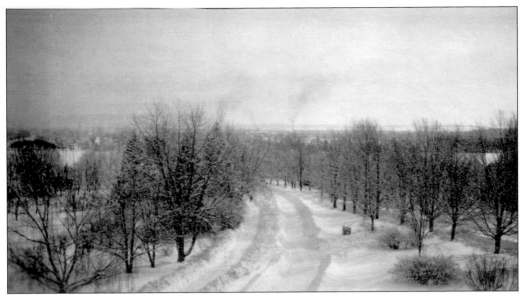

LOOKING TOWARD TOWN, 1927. This photograph from January of 1927 looks east from upstairs in Building 50 (above Hall 2), down 11th Street toward the intersection of 11th and Elmwood. Smoke rises from chimneys in the distance. (Courtesy of Julius Petertyl.)

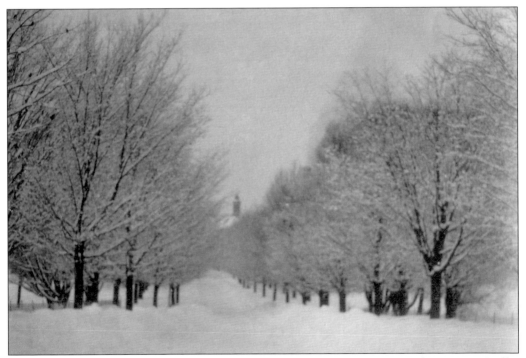

BUILDING 50, 1927. In this January 1927 photograph, the ventilation spire looms over Hall 2 of Building 50 in the distance. This view looks west from the intersection of 11th and Elmwood. (Courtesy of Julius Petertyl.)

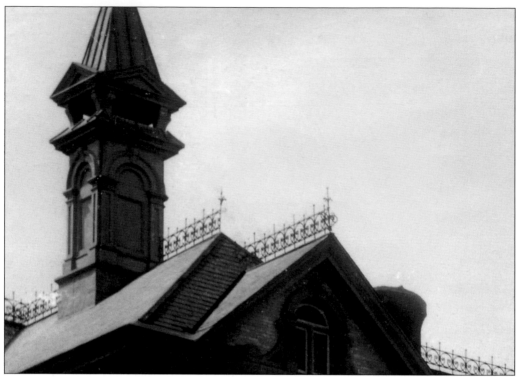

IRON RAILING ON ROOF. Iron railing such as that seen on the rooftop of Building 50 in this photograph was once a common architectural detail. This particular photograph is from the mid-20th century, and shows the roof and the first ventilation tower south of the center. This railing has been gone for decades. (Courtesy of George Beckett.)

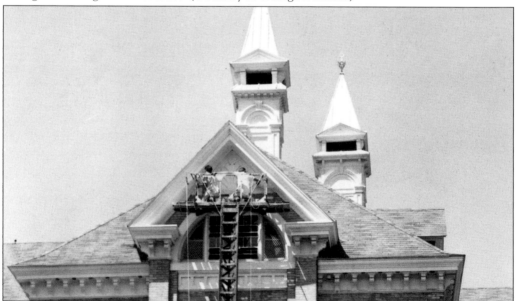

PAINTING THE EAVES, 1961. In this photo from 1961, painters atop a long wooden ladder work on the eaves of the northeast corner of Building 50. The paint on the bright white spires seen here was allowed to weather off after the building was closed.

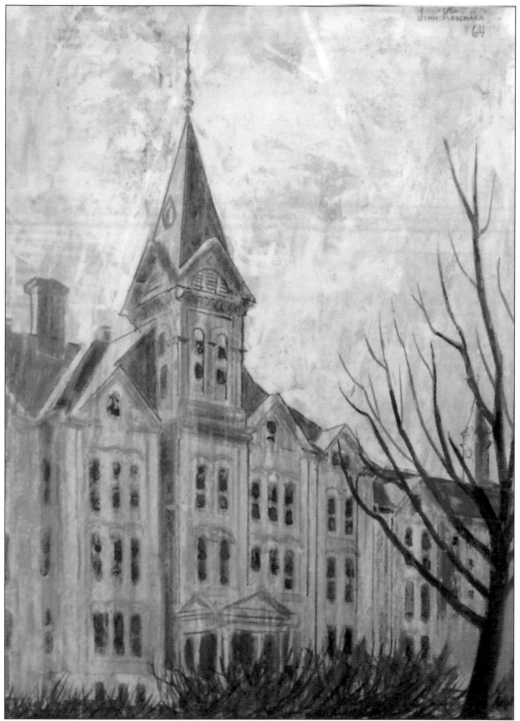

PAINTING OF OLD CENTER. This large painting has been in Building 50a (the new center) for many years. It was painted by John Koschara, and is dated 1964 (one year after this particular wing was demolished). It was donated in 1979 by Clifford Lindstrom. (Courtesy of the Grand Traverse Commons Redevelopment Corporation.)

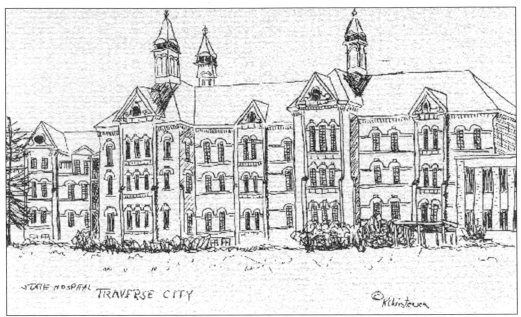

POSTCARD OF BUILDING 50, 1975. In 1975, artist Ken Christensen published this postcard of the front of the southern wing of Building 50 as part of a series of postcards of historic Traverse City buildings. These postcards were sold in area bookstores including Thompson News. Christensen was one of the first of the artists to rediscover the state hospital buildings and grounds. (Courtesy of Ken Christensen.)

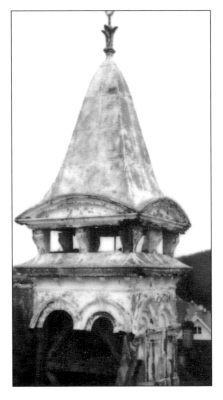

DAMAGED SPIRE, 1985. This photograph from November 21, 1985, shows the timbers framing the interior of the damaged spire on the south wing of Building 50. The front of this spire is currently covered to look like clapboard siding. (Courtesy of Paul Hansen.)

34

Three

MEN'S AND WOMEN'S COTTAGES

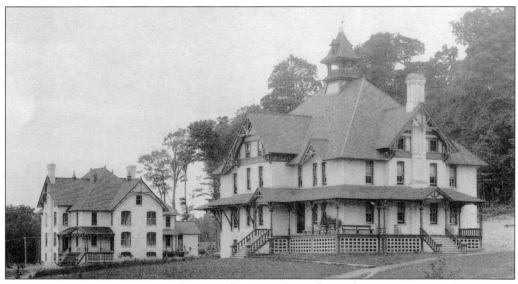

COTTAGES 32 AND 28. As Northern Michigan Asylum admitted more patients and grew more and more crowded, new buildings were constructed to house patients. This photo from shortly after construction shows Cottages A and B for men (now known as Cottages 32 and 28). The cottage buildings are presented in this chapter from north to south.

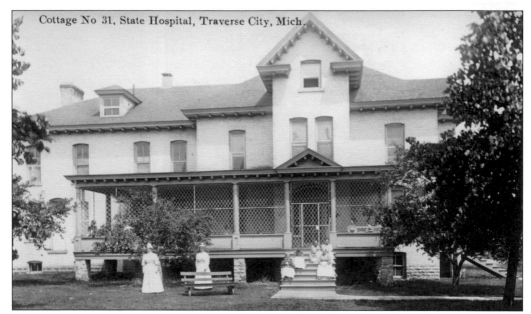

Cottage No 31, State Hospital, Traverse City, Mich.

COTTAGE 31. Cottage 31 was the northernmost of the state hospital cottages. Constructed in 1902, it was built for staff residence rather than for patient use. It was demolished mid-century to make room for medical hospital expansion (the only one of the historic brick cottages that has been lost). It was located near what is now the western wall of the Munson Tower section of Munson Hospital. (Courtesy of Heidi Johnson.)

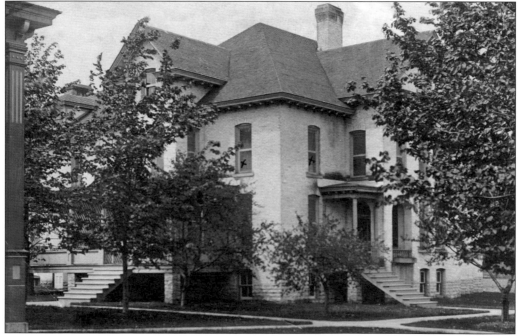

"SPENDING MY PRESENT DAYS." The writing on this photograph of Cottage 31 says, "Here's where I am spending my present days. Consumptive ward. Lovingly, Anna S. My room is where the sign X is in the windows." Consumptive is a word connected with tuberculosis. The view here is of the corner that is on the right in the first photograph on this page.

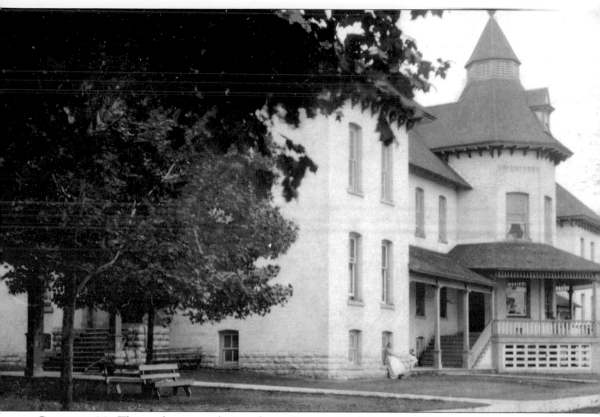

COTTAGE 29. This early postcard view shows Cottage 29. It is currently the northernmost of the cottage buildings. One of the women's cottages, it was built in 1893 and was a geriatric ward in its early years. Located just west of the Munson parking deck, it is currently mothballed. Aside from its covered windows, it still appears almost identical to what it was when this photograph was taken. (Courtesy of Julius Petertyl.)

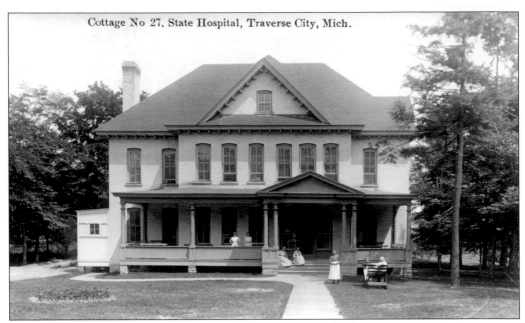

COTTAGE 27. Cottage 27 was built in 1903 as a residence for female patients. At one time, it was a ward for people with epilepsy. It is similar in plan to Cottage 36 in the southern (male) cottage group. It has been renovated as the Munson Hospitality House, which provides lodging for families of Munson Medical Center patients. (Courtesy of Heidi Johnson.)

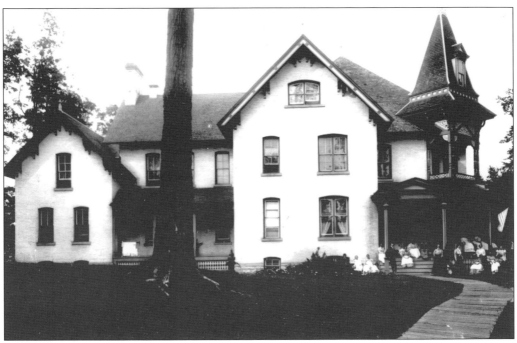

COTTAGE 25. The southeast-facing "Addams Family"-like tower of Cottage 25 has long since been removed, but there is still a corner porch. Constructed in 1891, this cottage served as a tuberculosis ward for female patients its early years. (Courtesy of the Grand Traverse Pioneer and Historical Society.)

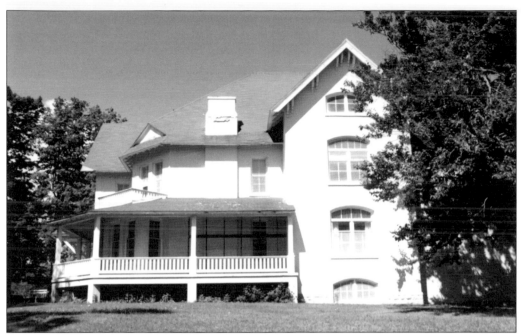

COTTAGE 25, 1986. This photograph from 1986 shows the eastern side of Cottage 25. From 1987 to 1991, this building served as the state hospital museum. Earle Steele was the curator. Part of Grand Traverse Pavilions, it was reopened in 2001 as assisted living senior apartments. It is now known as Willow Cottage. (Courtesy of Wigen, Tincknell, Meyer & Associates.)

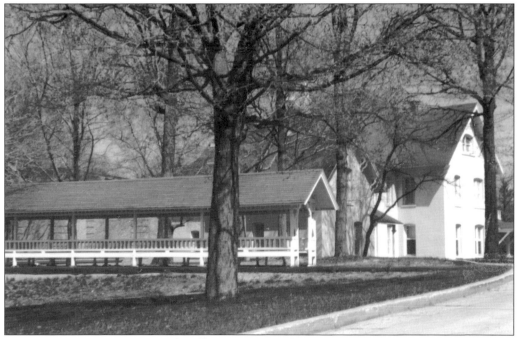

COVERED WALKWAYS. Covered walkways connected Cottage 27 to Building 39. These were demolished when Building 39 was removed in the mid-1990s. Seen here is the one that led to the south. Cottage 25 is behind it, to the right. (Courtesy of Julius Petertyl.)

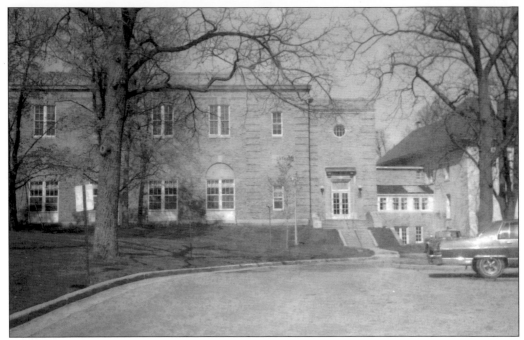

WOMEN'S AUDITORIUM. Building 39, constructed in 1924, was the women's dining hall, and also an auditorium. Its counterpart was Building 22 (the men's dining hall). This building was demolished in the mid-1990s to make way for Medical Campus Drive, which connected the medical campus to North Long Lake Road to the west. (Courtesy of Julius Petertyl.)

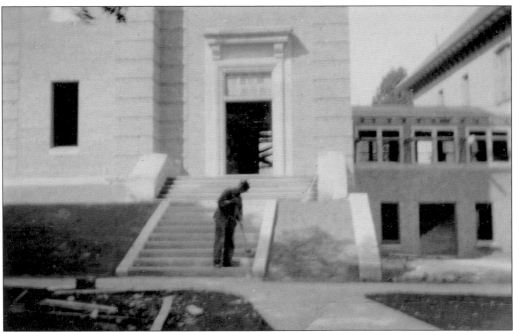

WOMEN'S AUDITORIUM UNDER CONSTRUCTION. Building 39, shown here toward the end of its construction, connected Cottages 25 and 29. Cottage 29 is seen on the right. (Courtesy of Julius Petertyl.)

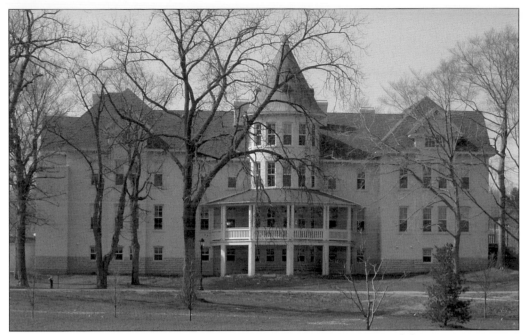

COTTAGE 23, 2003. Cottage 23 was built in the early 1900s as part of the women's cottage groups. It is connected via a one-story above-ground tunnel to Cottage 21, to the south. It was designed by C.S. Prahl. It is now known as Hawthorn Cottage (part of Grand Traverse Pavilions), and contains 26 studio and one bedroom apartments for older adults. It connects to the south to Cottage 21.

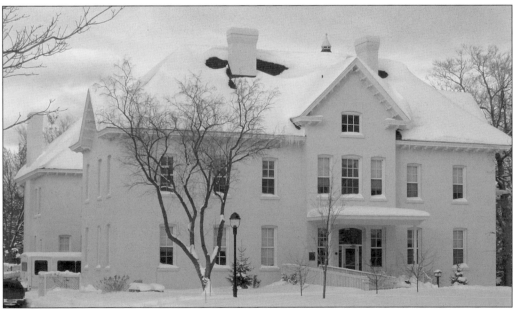

COTTAGE 21, "EVERGREEN COTTAGE." Cottage 21 was constructed in 1901. In its early years, it contained wards for female patients who worked in the asylum operations (such as laundry). It is now known as Evergreen Cottage, and is part of Grand Traverse Pavilions. This recent photo shows the south end, where it faces Building 50.

41

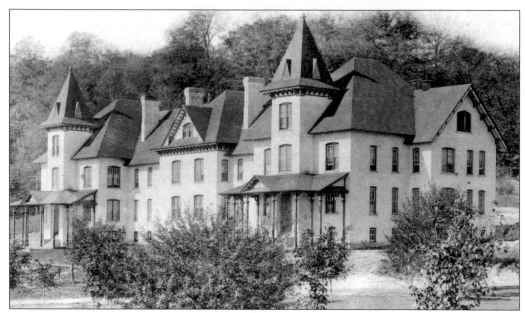

COTTAGE 40. Cottage 40 was built in 1893. This view from not long after its construction labels it "Cottage for Men," and the vantage point is from the southern rear courtyard of Building 50. It was also known as Cottages 24 and 26, and these other numbers are still found at one of the entrances. The first floor was at one time used as a hospital ward.

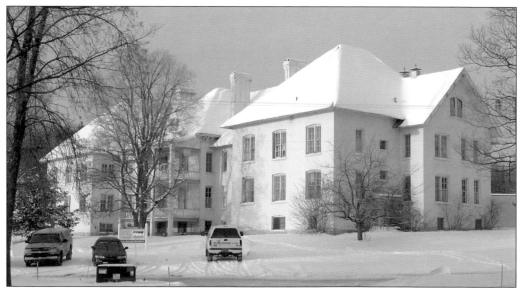

COTTAGE 40, 2004. Due to an alteration which removed the front towers and porches (and also added a porch in the center where there was none before), the front of Cottage 40 bears little resemblance to its original appearance. It is the northernmost of the men's cottages.

DOORBELLS OF COTTAGE 40, 2004. The doorbells at the rear entrance of Cottage 40 have two buttons, one for each floor. These labels refer to the building's alternate name of Cottage 24 and Cottage 26.

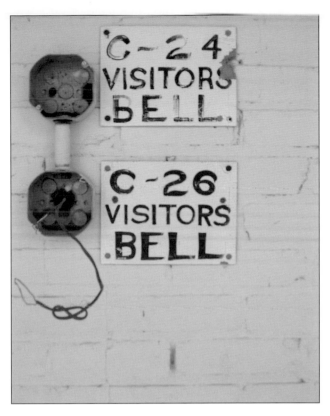

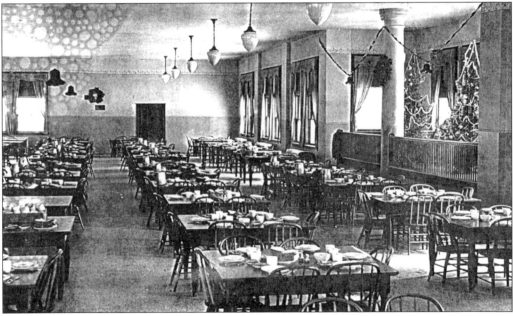

CHRISTMAS IN MEN'S CAFETERIA, 1925. A Christmas tree is seen set up on the right in this December 25, 1935 photo of the inside of the men's dining building (Building 22). This flat-roofed building was constructed in 1915 between Cottages 28 and 40. (Courtesy of the State Archives of Michigan.)

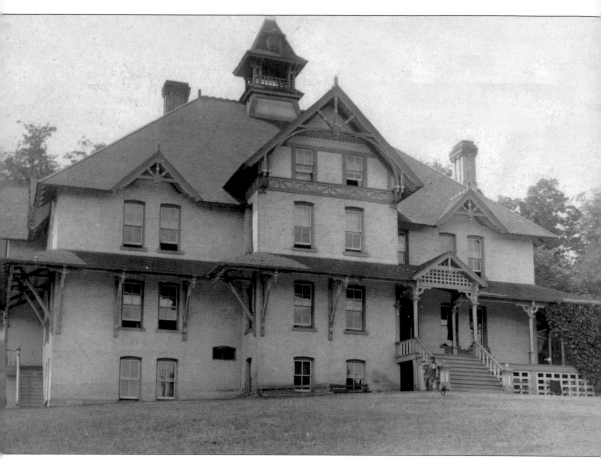

COTTAGE 28, FRONT. Cottage 28, constructed in the late 1880s, is unique among the cottages with its square shape and cupola. The wrap-around porch seen in this postcard photo from between 1904 and 1918 is long gone. This view is from the east lawn that is in front of the men's cottage buildings. (Courtesy of Julius Petertyl.)

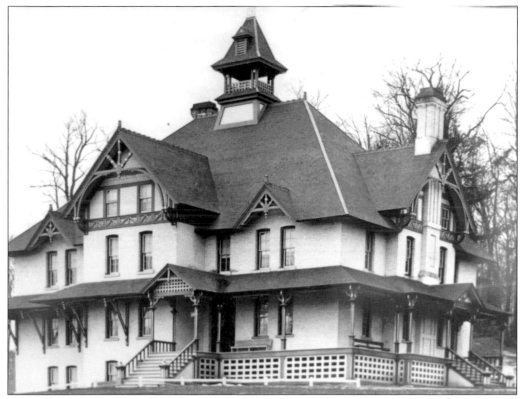

COTTAGE 28, CORNER. This vintage photograph shows the northeast corner of Cottage 28. The northern entrance seen on the right now adjoins Building 22. One of the uses of this building was to house geriatric patients.

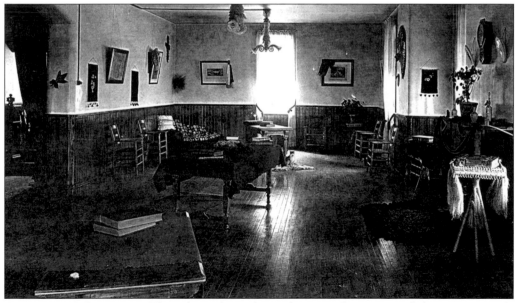

COTTAGE 28 INTERIOR. This photo from the early years shows one of the rooms inside Cottage 28. Note the desks and many books. (Courtesy of the State Archives of Michigan.)

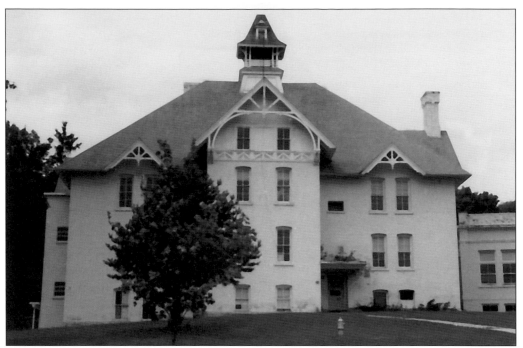

COTTAGE 28, 1986. Cottage 28 was one of the first to be abandoned. It looks much the same today. Part of Building 22 is seen on the right. A large dining hall for male patients, Building 22 connects to Cottage 40 on the north side. (Courtesy of Wigen, Tincknell, Meyer & Associates.)

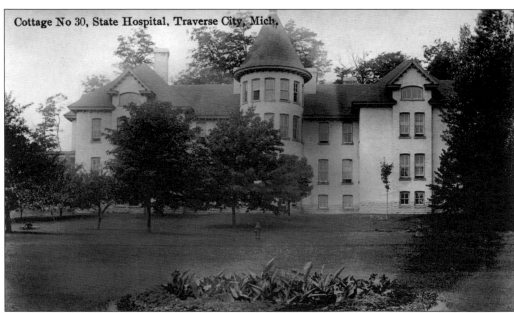

Cottage No 30, State Hospital, Traverse City, Mich,

COTTAGE 30, FRONT VIEW. Cottage 30 was built in 1901 to house male patients. This postcard view was produced between 1907 and 1929. In layout, Cottage 30 is very similar to Cottages 21 and 23, which also have east-facing round towers. This building looks much the same today. It is owned by the Minervini Group and is scheduled for renovation. (Courtesy of Heidi Johnson.)

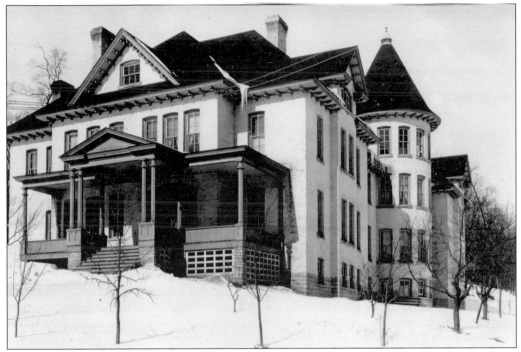

COTTAGE 30, SOUTHERN END. This photograph shows the southern end of Cottage 30. The dark-trimmed porch in this pre-1920s photograph of the south end was replaced later with a similar porch. (Courtesy of Julius Petertyl.)

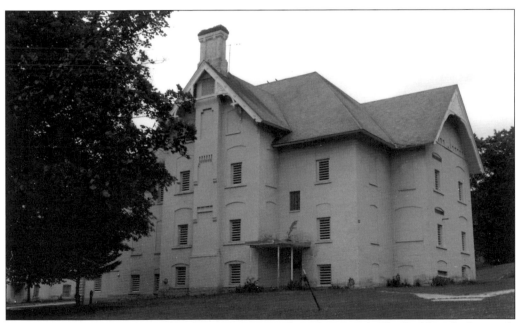

COTTAGE 32. Cottage 32 was built in 1889 as a tuberculosis ward. The building looks much the same today as it did in this 1986 photograph. The ornate porches from the early years (see the building on the left in the photo on p.35) have been removed and many of the windows are bricked in or blocked by security louvres. (Courtesy of Wigen, Tincknell, Meyer & Associates.)

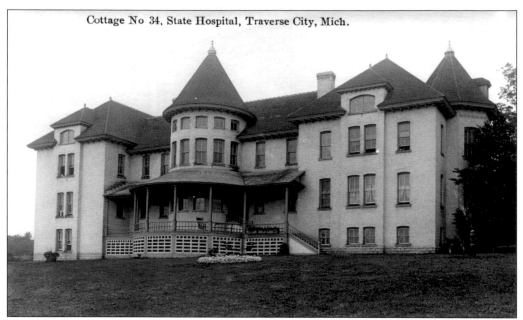

Cottage No 34, State Hospital, Traverse City, Mich.

COTTAGE 34. Cottage 34 was built in 1899 to house male patients who worked in the farms. It is also labeled "Hospital for Acute Insane (Men)" in old photographs. This postcard view of the building is from the first part of the 20th century. (Courtesy of Heidi Johnson.)

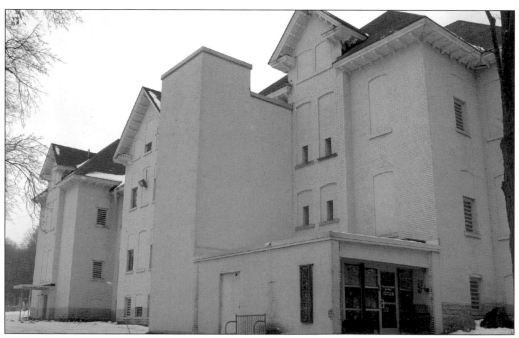

COTTAGE 36. This modern photo shows Cottage 36, which at one time housed patients who worked in the farms. It is very similar in plan to Cottage 27. This building has been in constant use, and now houses a day care center.

Four

BEAUTY IS THERAPY, WORK IS THERAPY
THE FARMS AND GROUNDS

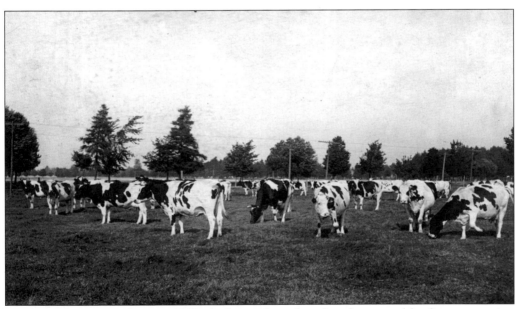

HERD OF HOLSTEINS. Late in 1885, the hospital purchased its first cows (the first one costing $20), along with a bull that cost $125. From this start, the state hospital built an outstanding dairy herd that at one time included a world champion milk cow. This chapter shows the history of the farms and the rest of the grounds.

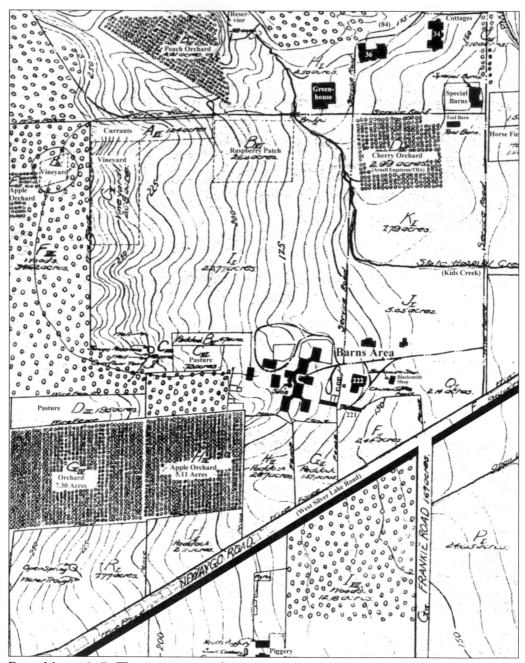

FARM MAP, 1917. This is a section of a surveyor's map of farm and grounds dating to 1917. For clarity, some buildings have been blackened, and some labels in a modern font have been added, as have some numbers for buildings for identification of still-standing structures. Some later features and names, not present yet in 1917, are identified in parentheses.

50

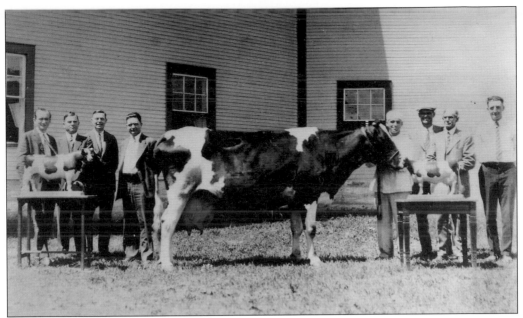

TRAVERSE COLANTHA WALKER. The state hospital herd at one time included a world champion milk cow named Traverse Colantha Walker. The cow's gravestone (located near the historic barns) reads, "Traverse Colantha Walker, 361604. Born 4-29-1916, Died 1-8-1932. World's Champion Cow. Milk: 200,114.9 lbs. Fat: 7,525 lbs. Nine Lactations. Bred, owned, developed by Traverse City Hospital."

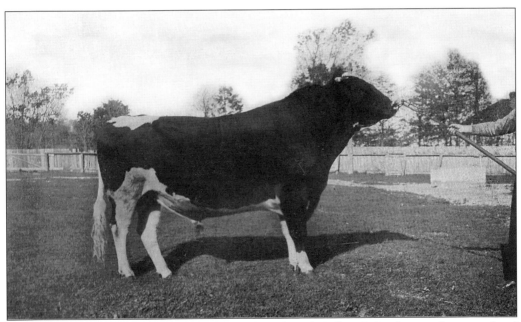

ADMIRAL WALKER. Another of the prize cattle, Admiral Walker Colantha was the senior herd sire. His weight at 3 years 10 months was 2300 lbs. The seven-day butter average of his four nearest dams was 32.83 lbs, and the 30-day average was 131.85 lbs. (Courtesy of the Grand Traverse Pioneer and Historical Society.)

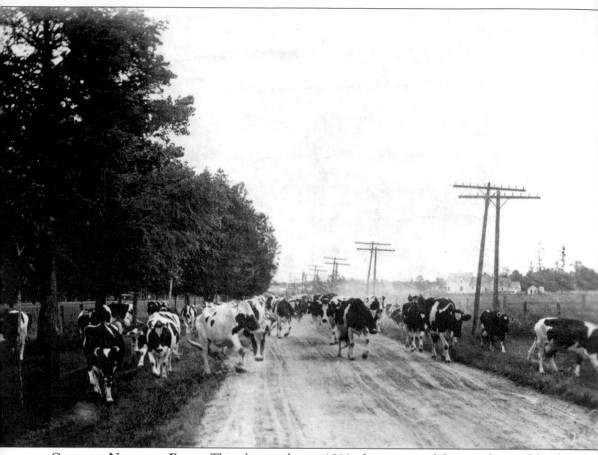

COWS ON NEWAYGO ROAD. This photo, taken c. 1911, shows cows of the state hospital herd headed west on what is now West Silver Lake Road. This road was once known as Newaygo Road. The building in the distance on the right was the residence of Ray Elliott (605 W. 14th). Ray Elliott was one of the attendants in Cottage 36. His residence is now the site of Tom's Supermarket at the southeast corner of 14th and Division.

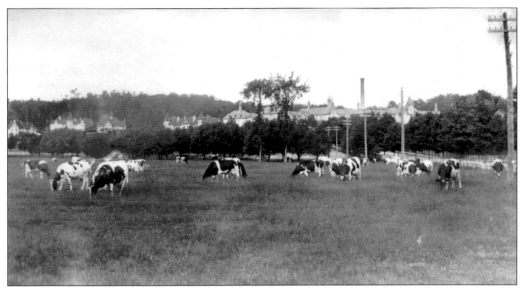

GRAZING HERD. In this photo, the herd grazes in pasturelands just south of Asylum Avenue (11th Street). This area is now grown over with trees, and is part of Sub-area 8 in the Grand Traverse Commons District Plan. This Sub-area is protected from development. (Courtesy of the State Archives of Michigan.)

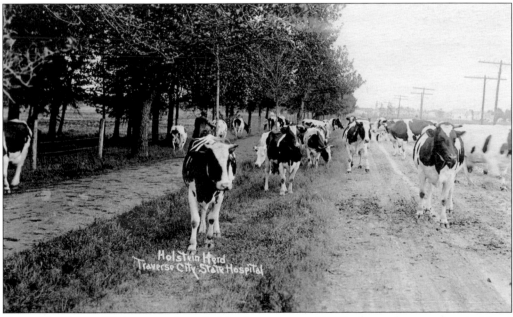

COWS ON ROAD. This postcard, mailed in the summer of 1926, shows the state hospital herd coming down one of the farm roads. Writing on the back of the postcard says, "Here we are milking the cows and fishing between times." A man with a bicycle with his back to the camera is behind the foremost cow. (Courtesy of George Beckett.)

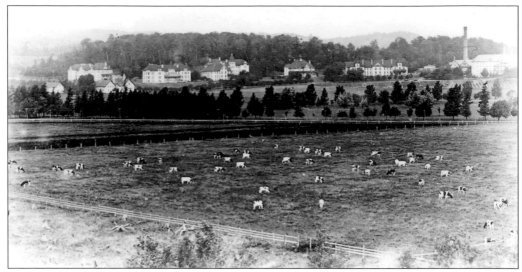

PASTURES. More than 50 head of Holstein cattle can be seen grazing in the pasture lands to the southeast of the state hospital buildings. The second building from the left is Cottage 36 with the "special barns" in front to the right. To the right (north) of this is Cottage 34, featuring a porch on the tower that is no longer there. Further to the left is Cottage 32, with Cottage 30 just behind it. Cottage 28 is alone in the center of the photo, followed by Cottage 40, and then Building 50 at the right edge. (Courtesy of the State Archives of Michigan.)

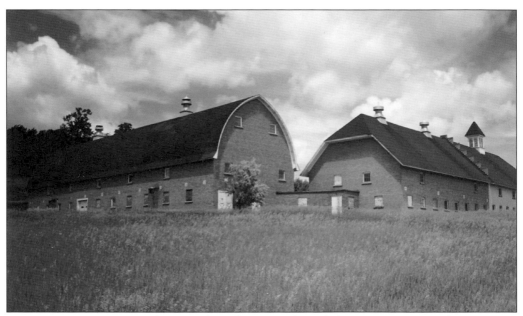

HISTORIC BARNS, 2001. These two large barns are the only barns remaining in the farm area. They were constructed in 1932 (left) and 1901 (right). An organization known as Rolling Centuries Historic Farm is working toward "rededicating them to recreational and educational goals." (Courtesy of the Grand Traverse Commons Redevelopment Corporation.)

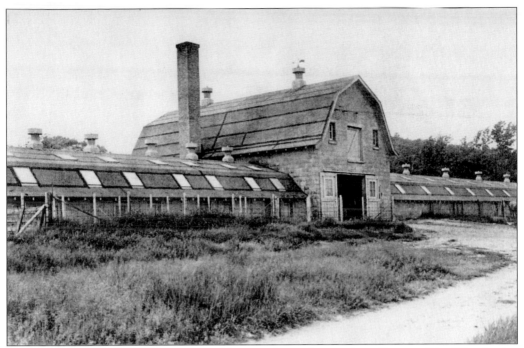

PIGGERY. The state hospital piggery building was located near where Traverse City West Junior High School is now, to the southwest of the Grand Traverse Commons grounds. Patients cared for the farm animals and did other farm work out of the belief that "work is therapy." (Courtesy of the Grand Traverse Commons Redevelopment Corporation.)

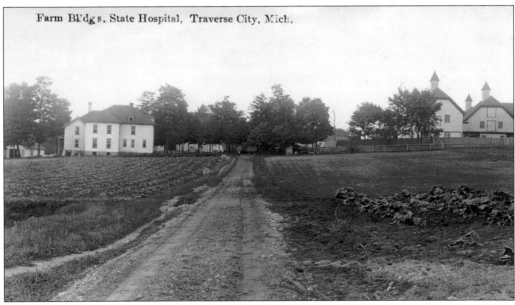

Farm Bl'dgs, State Hospital, Traverse City, Mich.

FARM BUILDINGS. This postcard, produced between 1907 and 1929, shows a view downSilver Drive from the north. Cottage 38 (demolished 1974) is on the left and the cow barns (demolished 1985) are on the right. Page 102 shows historic views in the other direction up Silver Drive. (Courtesy of Heidi Johnson.)

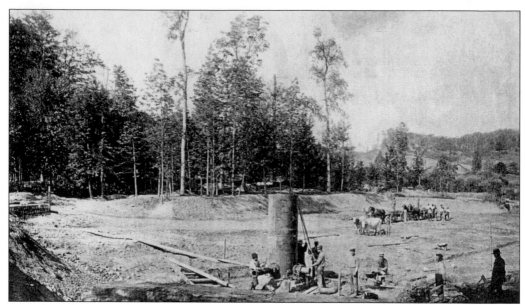

RESERVOIR UNDER CONSTRUCTION. Teams of oxen and horses and many men are shown here building the old reservoir. The farm work on the state hospital was done with animals well into the 1930s. (Courtesy of the Grand Traverse Commons Redevelopment Corporation.)

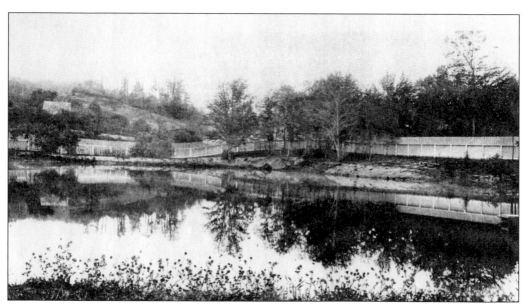

FENCED-IN RESERVOIR. The large hospital reservoir was located in the hills above (to the west) of the state hospital. The elevation ensured adequate water pressure and distribution to the state hospital. (Courtesy of the Grand Traverse Commons Redevelopment Corporation.)

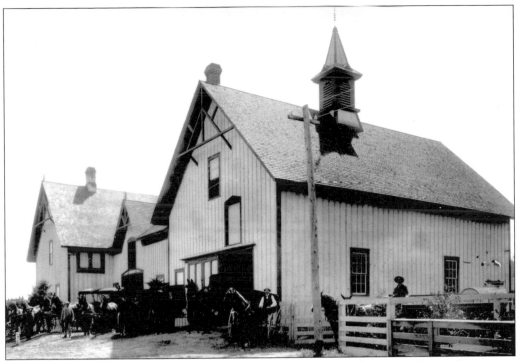

SPECIAL BARNS. The "Special Barns" were located to the east of Cottage 36 and the current site of the New Campus (Arnell Engstrom School). These buildings housed Dr. Munson's horse and buggy. As carriage houses were no longer needed, many were demolished, or turned into garages or residences. The carriage house for the steward's residence, at the northeast corner of the grounds, still stands. (Courtesy of the Grand Traverse Pioneer and Historical Society.)

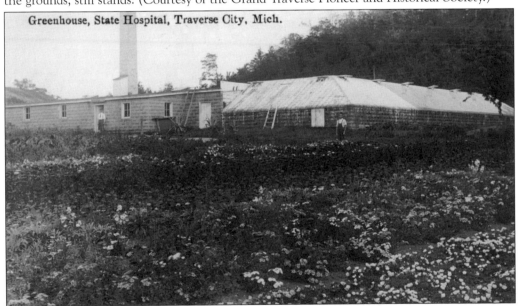

GREENHOUSE EXTERIOR. The extensive greenhouses provided food for the patients and productive work. The greenhouses were located west of what is now the Traverse Bay Area Intermediate School District administration building, between the barns and Building 50.

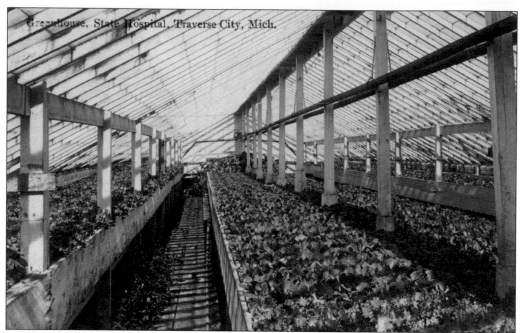

INSIDE THE GREENHOUSE. Among the plants grown in the greenhouses were flowers thatwere distributed to the wards to beautify them.

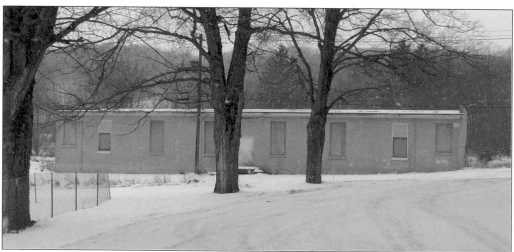

BUILDING 44. All that remains of the old greenhouse complex is the concrete block building that attached the east ends of the actual greenhouses. Currently designated Building 44, this building is scheduled to be renovated and expanded and opened as Greenspire Montessori School in 2005. "A Montessori junior high dedicated to the great work of the adolescent," Greenspire emphasizes agricultural and natural education. This particular view shows the front (east side) of the building. The greenhouses were behind, in what is now a flat grassy area.

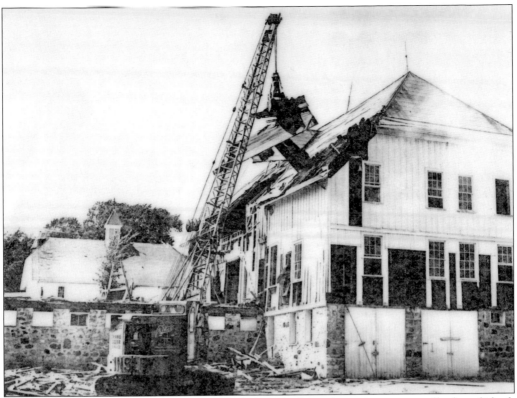

HORSE BARN. All of the wooden barns, including the horse barn, were eventually demolished. After the wooden upper structure was demolished, the lower stone foundation section was kept for storage use. (Courtesy of the State Archives of Michigan.)

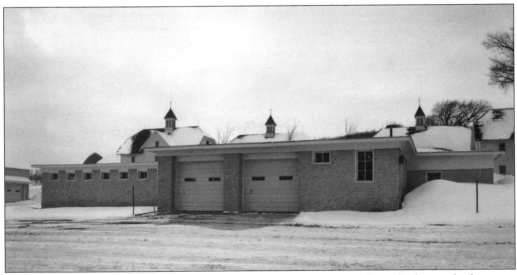

BUILDING 222. Building 222, the basement of the former horse barn, looks much the same today as it did in this vintage photograph from before the wooden cow barns (seen in the background) were removed in the 1970s. This building has been used for storage. (Courtesy of Paul Hansen.)

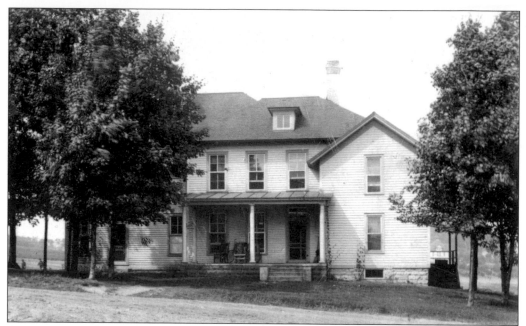

COTTAGE 38. This was located near the barns. Constructed in 1900, it was demolished in 1974 along with the rest of the wooden buildings in the farm area of the state hospital grounds. It was used to house patients who worked in the farm. This photo is from between 1904 and 1918. (Courtesy of Julius Petertyl.)

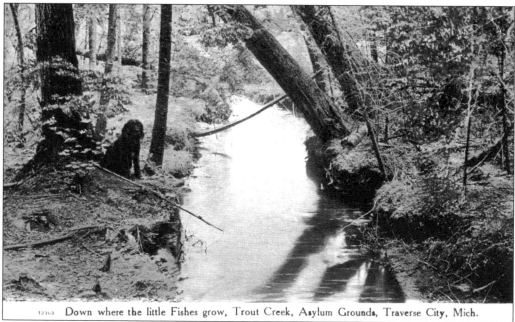

12363 Down where the little Fishes grow, Trout Creek, Asylum Grounds, Traverse City, Mich.

"DOWN WHERE THE LITTLE FISHES GROW." The postcard shown here, mailed in 1911, is one of two different ones that show a dog alongside the creek in the state hospital grounds. The stream flows from south of Traverse City through the state hospital grounds and into the Boardman River west of downtown Traverse City. At one time called Mill Creek, it later became Asylum Creek, and is now known as Kids Creek.

LOVER'S LANE. Lover's Lane ran west from Division Street to Elmwood and beyond. The path was made of cinders from the power plant. This was a popular place for families to take a stroll on Sundays. Much of it was removed in the 1950s, when trees were chopped down. Today, there is a "Women's Walk" near where Lover's Lane used to run.

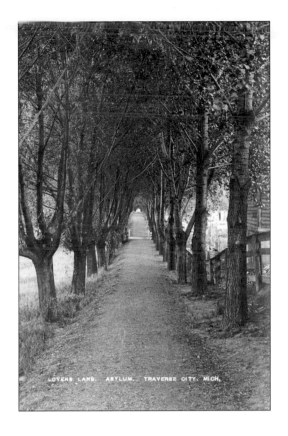

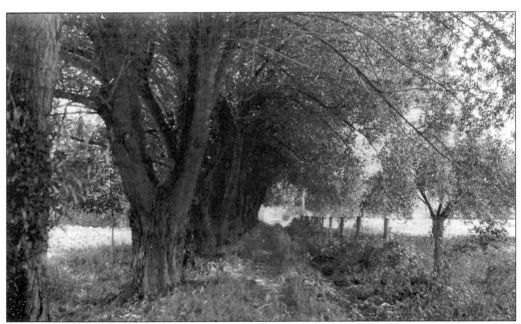

LOVER'S LANE, 1925. This postcard view from 1925 shows Lover's Lane, as seen looking west from the back of the residence at 717 West 7th Street. (Courtesy of Julius Petertyl.)

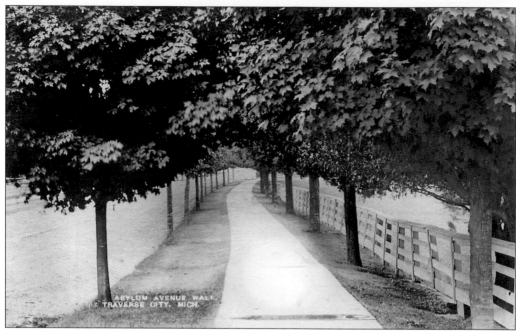

ASYLUM AVENUE. Asylum Avenue is an earlier name for the western end of 11th Street. This vintage photo shows a tree-shadowed sidewalk along the gently winding avenue. (Courtesy of George Beckett.)

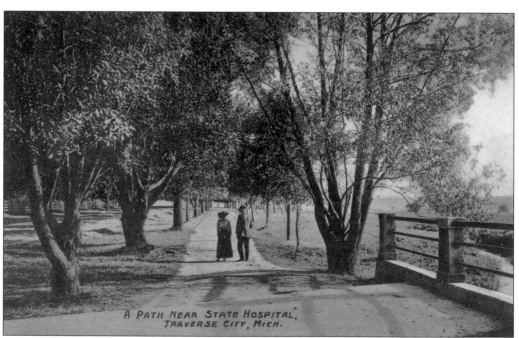

PATH. This postcard was signed on the back by its creator, Orson W. Peck: "This shows myself and my southern friend, taking the photo myself with a thread." (Courtesy of George Beckett.)

FOUR WOMEN AT GATE. Four women stand at the Elmwood gate, c. 1914. From the left are Irene Pike (daughter of steward George Pike), Edith Hurt, Irene Petertyl, and Anna Turek. All but the first are cousins of Julius Petertyl. Julius Petertyl lived across the street from the hospital grounds, and was a brickmason who worked on several of the buildings. (Courtesy of Julius Petertyl.)

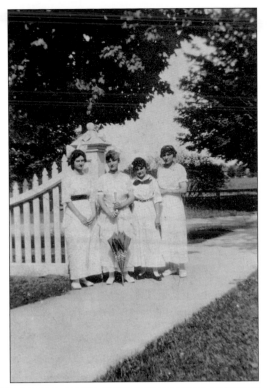

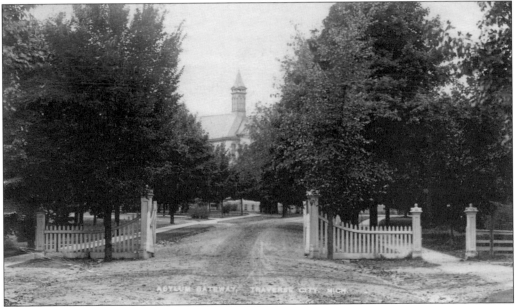

ELMWOOD GATE. This postcard, mailed in 1910, shows the main Elmwood Avenue gate, at the west end of Asylum Avenue (11th Street). One of the captions in the state hospital calendar from 1974 read, "Those fences were an indicator of the philosophy of institutions for the mentally ill to keep people in. They were likewise indicators of the fear of the community outside. These fences have come down and the new philosophy of a much better understanding of care and treatment has changed the life and the hope for the patient."

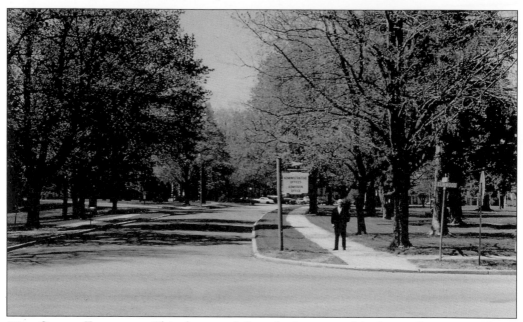

11TH STREET ENTRANCE. This photograph from the last years of the hospital's operation shows where the main gate used to stand. The view is similar, but not identical to that in the 1910 postcard view (the spire is hidden by the trees). The arrow part of the sign, which pointed toward the administration building, still remains. (Courtesy of Julius Petertyl.)

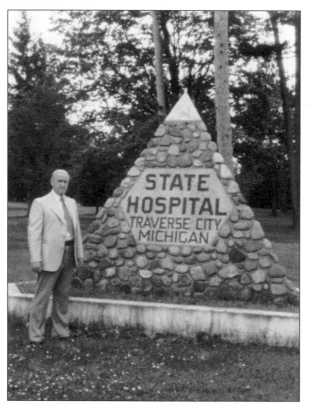

PYRAMID BUILDER, 1985. In this photo from May 12, 1985, Paul Hansen stands next to the stone pyramid he and David Levinski built in the summer of 1965. The future of this pyramid was in doubt during the 1990s, and the letters naming the state hospital were chiseled off. Now it stands with wooden plaques that welcome visitors to Traverse City. (Courtesy of Paul Hansen.)

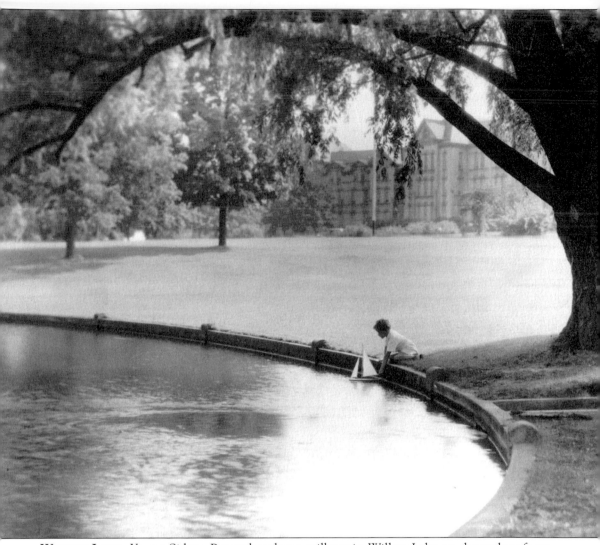

WILLOW LAKE. Young Sidney Petertyl pushes a sailboat in Willow Lake on the asylum front lawn in this photograph from 1933 or 1934. This photograph was taken by his father, Willard Petertyl. The Petertyls lived in Traverse City's Central Neighborhood, just east of the state hospital grounds across Division Street. (Courtesy of Julius Petertyl.)

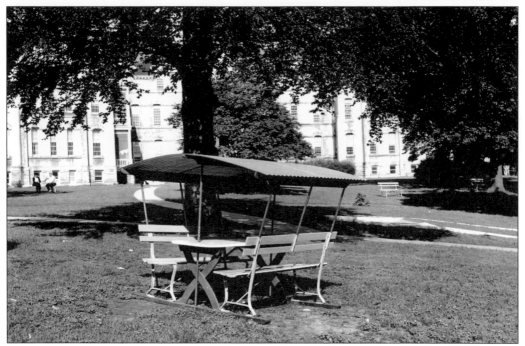

PICNIC TABLE ON FRONT LAWN. The picnic table seen in front of Building 50 in this photo from the 1960s or 1970s was made in the state hospital carpenter shop. Workers in the shop repaired broken furniture and built new furniture, like this table. (Courtesy of Paul Hansen.)

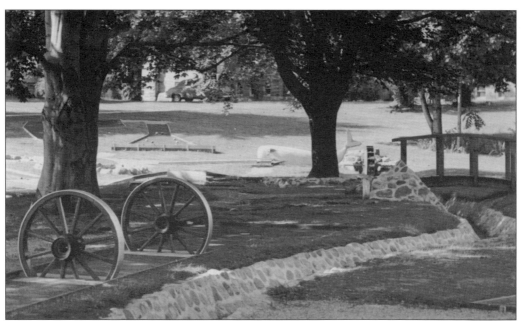

MINIATURE GOLF COURSE. A miniature golf course on the front lawn between Building 50 and Willow Lake provided recreational opportunities for patients and staff. A white whale can be seen behind the tree to the right of center, and a waterwheel is behind the whale's tail. The golf course was removed during the superintendency of Dr. Philip B. Smith. (Courtesy of Paul Hansen.)

Five

OTHER BUILDINGS

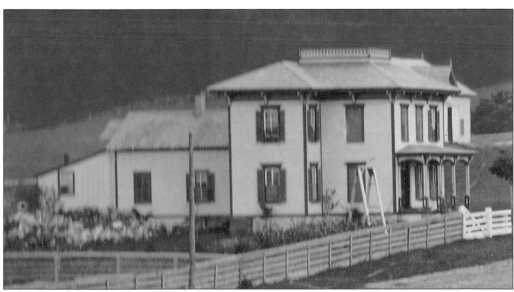

ORIGINAL FARMHOUSE, 1884. In addition to the main patient housing and farm buildings, many other buildings were needed in the operation of the hospital. Depicted here is the first building on the grounds during the time of the construction of Building 50. (Courtesy of the Con Foster Museum.)

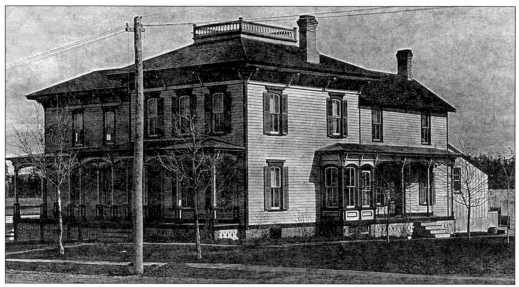

FARMHOUSE. The white wooden building now known as "Old Munson Hall" (Building 88) is the oldest building at Grand Traverse Commons, and is one of the oldest buildings in Traverse City. It was built as a farmhouse in 1879 before Northern Michigan Asylum was founded. In the early years of the institution, it served as a ward for female patients. (Courtesy of the State Archives of Michigan.)

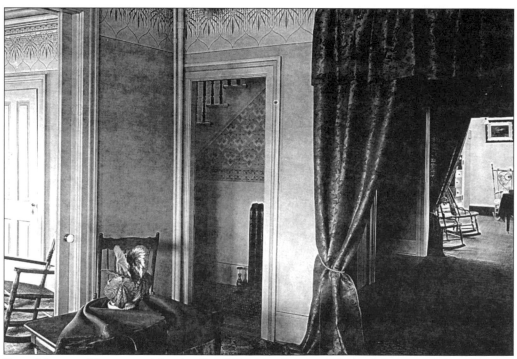

FIRST MUNSON HOSPITAL. After the Grand Traverse Sanitarium burned down in 1915, Building 88 became the first Munson Hospital, serving Traverse City's general medical needs. It was later used as staff apartments. The layout of the rooms on the first floor (now used for private offices) has changed a lot since this early photo was taken. (Courtesy of the State Archives of Michigan.)

Steward's Residence c. 1973. The steward's residence was located at the far northeast corner of the grounds. It was authorized in the 1896 report by the asylum board of trustees: "As we deemed it highly important that the steward should reside on the asylum grounds, it was decided to build a house for his use. The residence is located at the corner of Eighth and Division Streets. It is an eight-room, two-story frame building and it is supplied with water and light from the asylum. Its cost, complete, is about $2,500." In 1973, when this photo was taken, it housed the director of research and training. It was recently sold to a private owner who put a lot of work into restoring it. (Courtesy of Julius Petertyl.)

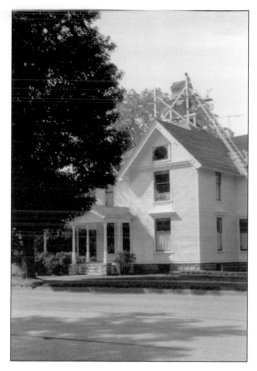

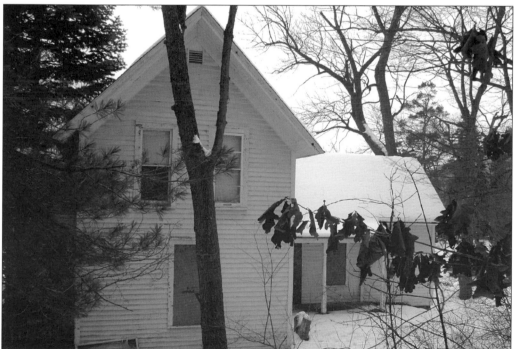

Gardener's House, 2004. This wooden house located to the west of Cottage 36 was constructed in 1890 as an engineer's residence. Later, it became the gardener's house. Earl Steele grew up here. It has long been vacant. One of the future uses discussed for this house has been to turn it into a brew-pub.

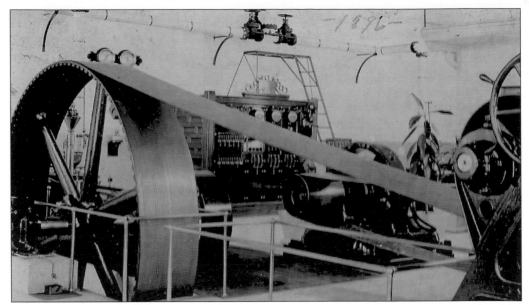

POWER PLANT. This photo shows the machines inside the original power plant in 1896. The small sign seen beneath the valves and ladder at the center top is now on display at the Grand Traverse Heritage Center. It says, "Northern Michigan Asylum—Installed by General Electric Co, 1896." (Courtesy of the Grand Traverse Pioneer and Historical Society.)

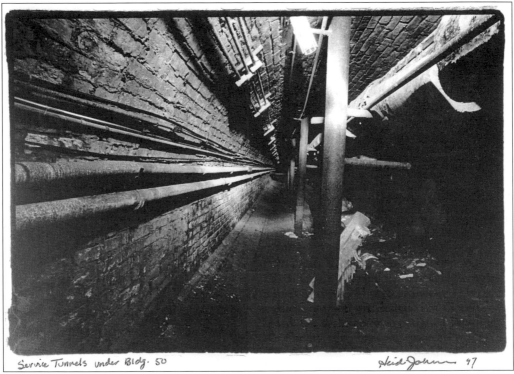

Service Tunnels under Bldg. 50

Heidi Johnson 97

STEAM TUNNEL. There are many tunnels connecting the buildings of the former state hospital. Some are walkable, others can only be crawled. Some have utilities, and some do not. The tunnels were never used for housing patients. (Photograph by Heidi Johnson.)

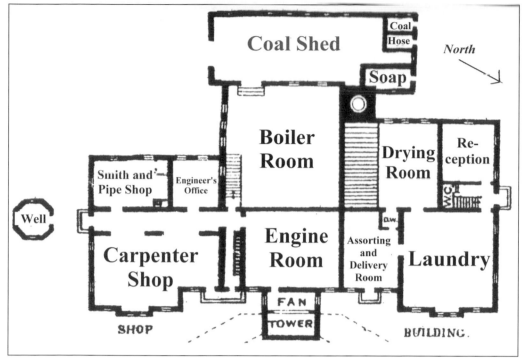

SHOP BUILDING FLOOR PLAN. This floor plan shows the original shop building and the uses of its different sections. It was constructed in 1893 and demolished in the 1940s. It was immediately behind (to the west of) the chapel wing. The shop building, with its 150-foot smokestack, can be seen behind Building 50 in the air photos on pages 107 and 108.

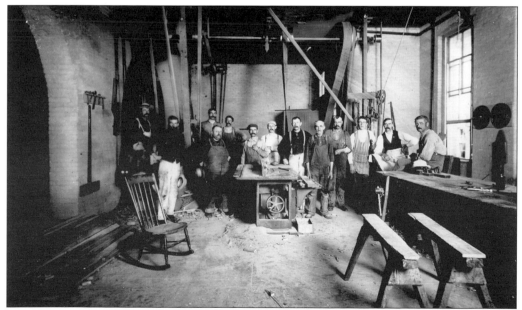

OLD CARPENTRY SHOP. The carpenters pose for a photo in the old carpentry shop during the early days of the state hospital. The shop was in the southeast corner of the original shop building. (Courtesy of the Grand Traverse Pioneer and Historical Society.)

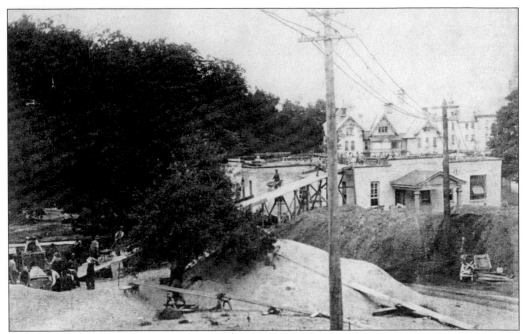

CONSTRUCTION OF OLD LAUNDRY BUILDING, 1890S. The old laundry building was constructed in the 1890s. It was located in front of the current laundry building location. It was one of many service buildings to the back of the center of Building 50. It was demolished in the 1940s. Hall 19 is in the background on the right. (Courtesy of the State Archives of Michigan.)

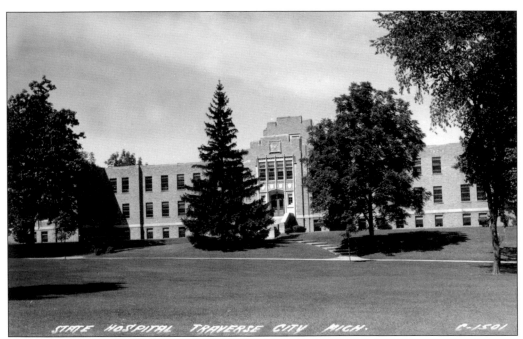

BUILDING 33, 1930S. Building 33 was constructed in 1930, west of the similar (but not identical) Building 35. It started out as a TB (tuberculosis) ward (one of four buildings specifically for this purpose during the state hospital's history).

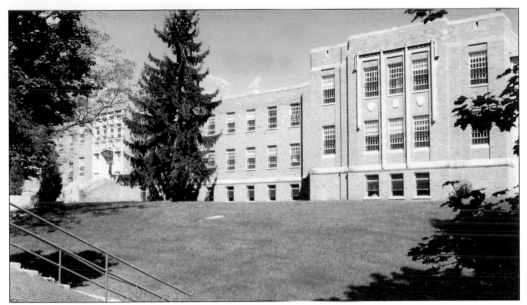

BUILDING 33, 1986. This photo from 1986 shows the south façade of Building 33. Building 33, along with its two other neighbor "flat top" buildings, was determined to be a building that could not be adapted to new usage, and it was demolished in the mid-1990s. (Courtesy of Wigen, Tincknell, Meyer & Associates.)

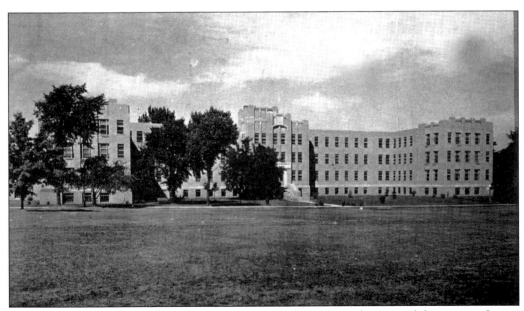

BUILDING 35, 1937. Building 35 was constructed in 1930. At the time of this postcard view (mailed in 1937), it was a children's clinic. It also served as an infirmary at one time.

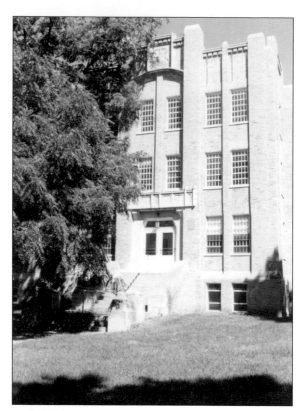

BUILDING 35, 1986. This photo from 1986 shows the entrance section of Building 35. The style of the ornamentation near the entrance is similar to that seen on the other 1930s-era buildings. (Courtesy of Wigen, Tincknell, Meyer & Associates.)

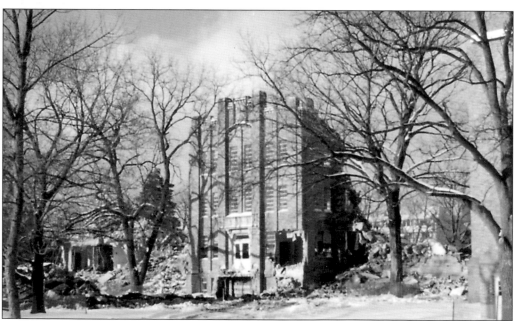

BUILDING 35 DEMOLISHED, 1995. Over the years, uses of Building 35 included being an outpatient clinic and housing geriatric patients. In the winter of 1995–1996, it was demolished to make way for the construction of Grand Traverse Pavilions. This photo shows the front entrance during demolition. (Courtesy of the Grand Traverse Commons Redevelopment Corporation.)

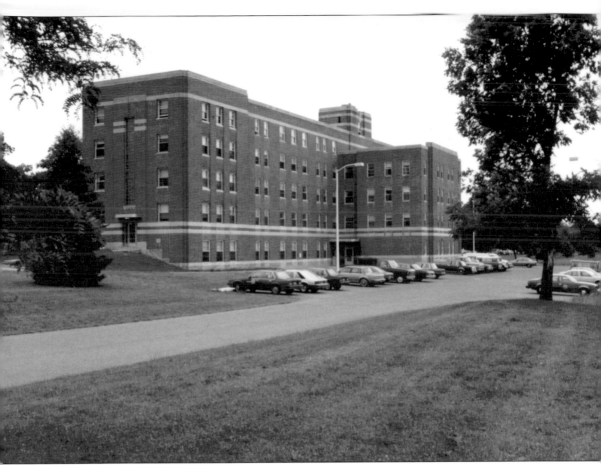

Employees' Building. Building 42 today looks much as it did when it was built in 1938, except for upgrading to more efficient windows and the addition of another story on the rear wing of the building. The extra story was added after this photograph from 1986 was taken. It was constructed as housing for nurses and other employees. This building is now a state office building, and houses several agencies of the State of Michigan.

The entry from the State Hospital Employee's Handbook (late 1960s) reads:

> *This hospital has a rather large and modern Employees' Building. There is often a waiting list for rooms there. If you are interested in living there, you should see the supervisor of that Building and request that she put your name on the waiting list for a room. All of the employees who live in the Employees' Building are adults, therefore, we have not published an extensive list of rules of conduct for those living there.*

(Courtesy of Wigen, Tincknell, Meyer & Associates.)

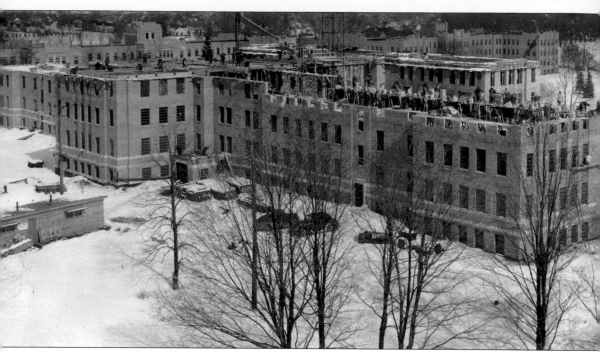

BUILDING 37 UNDER CONSTRUCTION, 1939. Building 37, the receiving hospital, was built in the late 1930s. The engineering and architectural firm was Shreve, Anderson and Walker of Detroit. The contracting company was H.G. Christman of Lansing. The Christman Company's recent projects include the renovation of the Michigan State Capitol building. Buildings 33 and 35 are in the background, and West Grand Traverse Bay is in the far distance. (Courtesy of Julius Petertyl.)

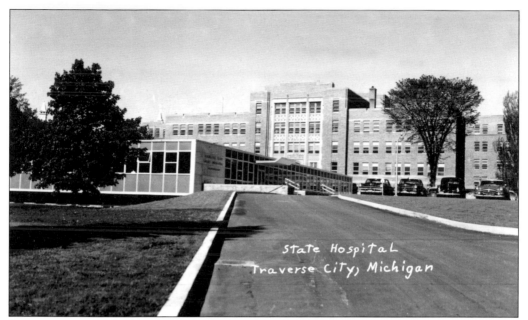

BUILDING 37. As the hospital's operations wound down, more and more of its operations were transferred to Building 37 and Building 37a. (Courtesy of George Beckett.)

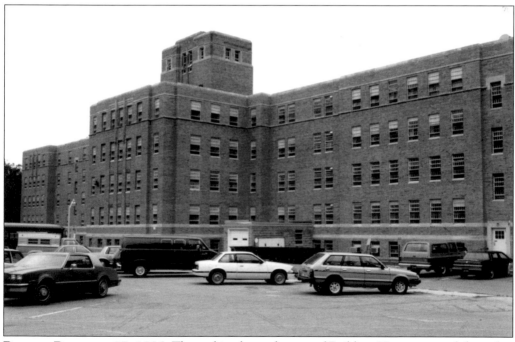

REAR OF BUILDING 27, 1986. The parking lot at the rear of Building 37 was accessed through a driveway that ran between the north end of Building 50 and Cottage 21. The driveway has been restored to lawn, and much of this parking lot was planted with grass and trees after the Grand Traverse Pavilions were completed. (Courtesy of Wigen, Tincknell, Meyer & Associates.)

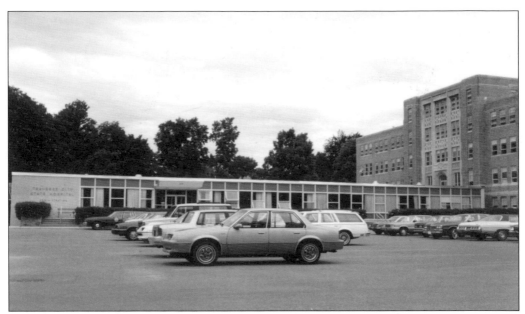

BUILDING 37A, 1986. Constructed in 1957, Building 37a was attached to the front of the receiving hospital, Building 37. This was the administration section during the hospital's last years. This wing was demolished along with the rest of Building 37 in the mid 1990s to make way for the construction of Grand Traverse Pavilions. (Courtesy of Wigen, Tincknell, Meyer & Associates.)

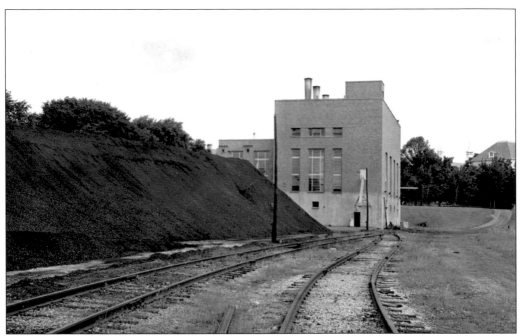

NEW POWER PLANT. The new power plant was built in 1948 south of Building 50. First powered by coal delivered by rail, later, it was converted to burn fuel oil. Two yellow fuel tanks now stand to the south of the building. (Courtesy of the Grand Traverse Pioneer and Historical Society.)

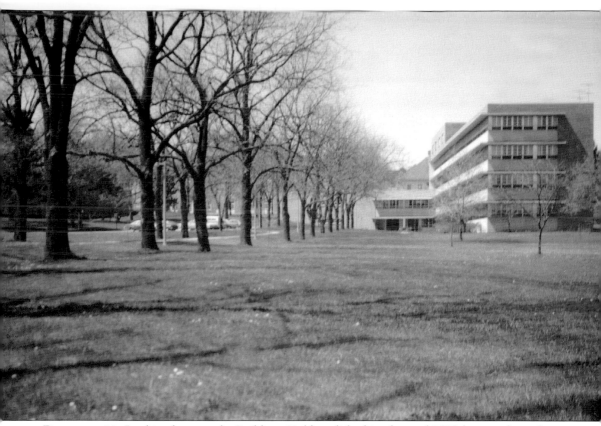

BUILDING 41. In this photograph, Building 41 (demolished in the mid-1990s) is on the right, and the western end of the tree-lined Lover's Lane is on the left. Building 41 was the last building constructed as a TB ward. During its last years, it was used for housing geriatric patients. The Munson Hospital parking deck now stands on this site. (Courtesy of Julius Petertyl.)

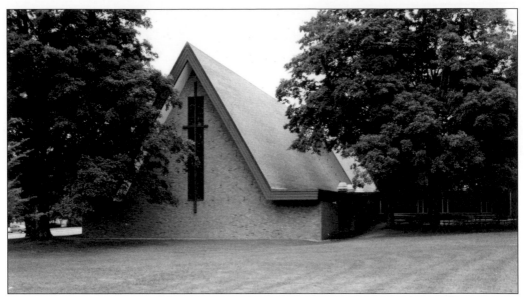

ALL FAITHS CHAPEL. The All Faiths Chapel was constructed in 1963 on the northwest corner of 11th and Elmwood Streets. This was a special project of superintendent Dr. M. Duane Somerness and others to meet the worship needs of the patients. The building was constructed with a Protestant sanctuary on one end, a Catholic sanctuary on the other, and a small synagogue in the middle. (Courtesy of Wigen, Tincknell, Meyer & Associates.)

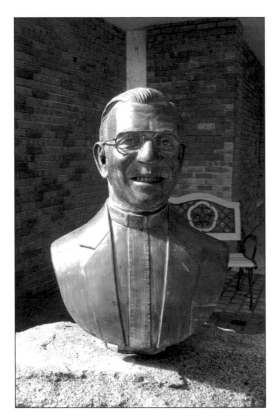

BUST OF "FATHER FRED," 2004. The All Faiths Chapel building today looks much as it did when it was built, but it is no longer a place of worship. It currently houses non-profit agencies. A bust of Father Erwin J. Frederick (1925–2000), who served as state hospital chaplain for 31 years, stands by the entrance. He was beloved figure in Traverse City State Hospital and the community. "Father Fred" founded the "Father Fred Foundation," a community charity that has provided clothing, food, and other items to thousands of families.

Six

MUNSON HOSPITAL AND RELATED PLACES

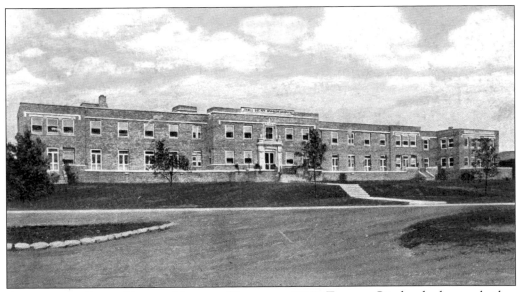

POSTCARD OF JAMES DECKER MUNSON HOSPITAL, 1929. Traverse City has had several other hospitals and custodial care institutions over the years. Munson Medical Center, which was started by Dr. James Decker Munson as part of Traverse City State Hospital, is now the primary provider of medical services for the region.

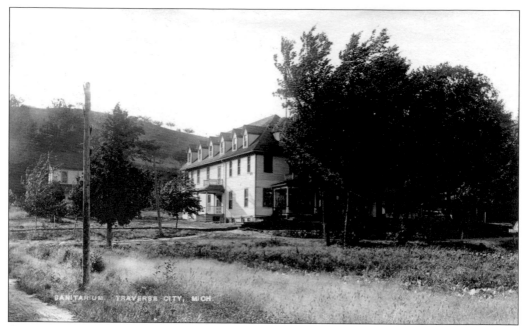

GRAND TRAVERSE SANITARIUM, 1900S. One of the earliest hospitals in the area was established in 1901 in Elmwood Township by Dr. Victor H. Sturm. It was located where Tom's West Bay shopping center is now located. Fire destroyed it in 1915, creating a medical care need in the community which Dr. Munson answered by turning Building 88 into a hospital.

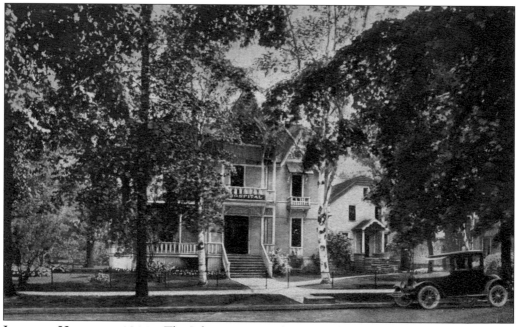

JOHNSON HOSPITAL, 1910S. The Johnson Hospital, seen in this postcard from the 1910s, was located on the southeast corner of State and Wellington. A cluster of small stucco houses now stands on the site.

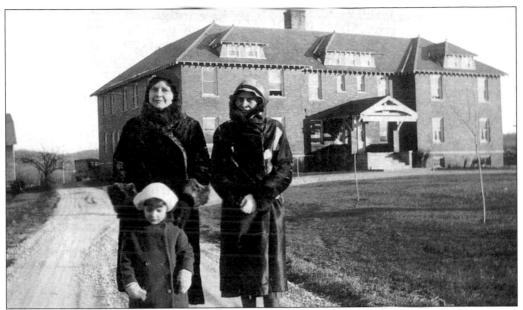

BOARDMAN VALLEY HOSPITAL, 1930s. Boardman Valley Hospital was built as Grand Traverse County's poorhouse in 1911. Over the years it evolved into a medical care facility. It was rendered obsolete by the construction of Grand Traverse Medical Care near Munson Hospital in 1959. This photo shows the hospital in the early 1930s. The adults (left to right) are Gladys Mielke and Adeline Mielke. The little girl is Mickey (Mielke) Thomas. The building faced west to Cass Road. The Boardman river valley was behind it. (Courtesy of Larry Wakefield.)

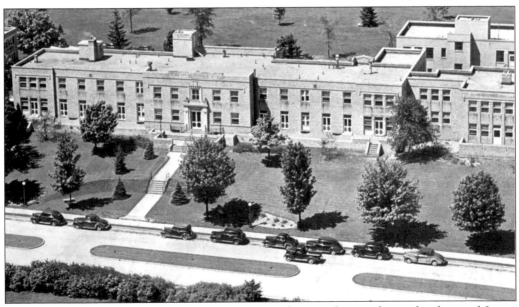

AERIAL VIEW OF MUNSON HOSPITAL, 1920s. This aerial view shows the front of James Decker Munson Hospital (facing east), completed in 1925. It had 25 beds at the time. The annex can be seen at the far left edge. The annex was a state hospital building that was used for nursing education. It was later absorbed into Munson Hospital, but it still juts out from the rear southwestern corner of the hospital. (Courtesy of Julius Petertyl.)

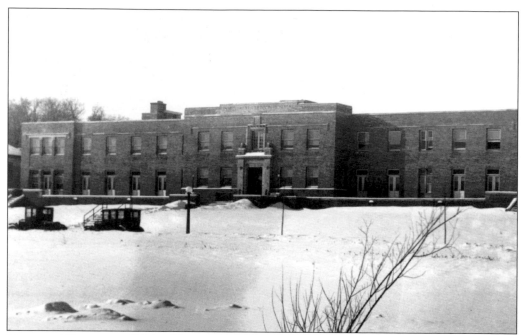

MUNSON HOSPITAL, 1920s. This postcard photo shows the front of James Decker Munson Hospital shortly after it was constructed. The name of the hospital is etched in the concrete at the top of the wall above the center entrance.

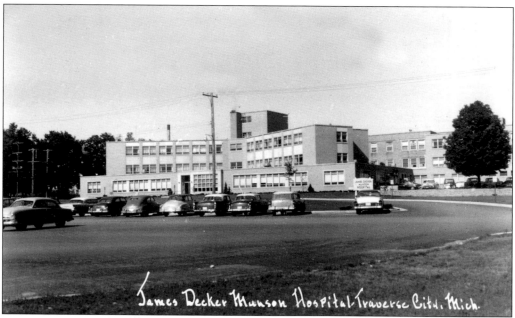

MUNSON HOSPITAL, 1950s. This postcard view from the 1950s shows James Decker Munson Hospital, looking southwest across the parking lot. The original building can be seen to the right, behind the newer Y-shaped wing.

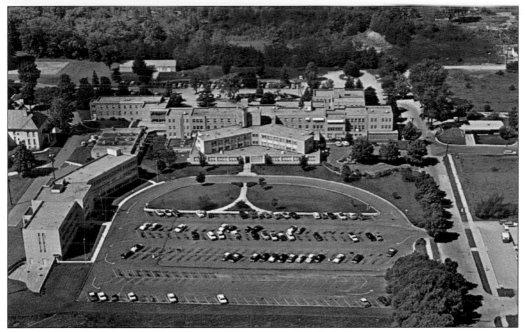

MUNSON HOSPITAL, 1960S. This chrome-era postcard shows an aerial view of Munson Hospital from the late 1960s. The angled building in the lower left is Grand Traverse Medical Care, and the peak-roofed building at the center left edge is Building 29, the northernmost building of Traverse City State Hospital. (Courtesy of Phil Balyeat.)

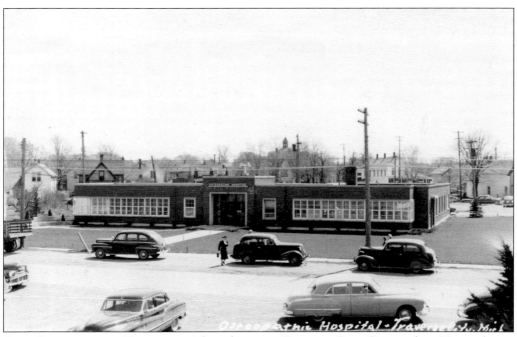

OLD OSTEOPATHIC HOSPITAL. After the new Traverse City Osteopathic Hospital was constructed, its previous building was renovated and dedicated as a lodge of the Benevolent and Protective Order of Elks in July of 1965. It remains as Elks Lodge No. 323 to this day.

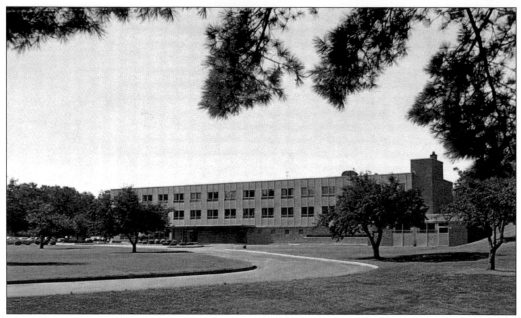

NEW OSTEOPATHIC HOSPITAL BUILDING. In 1962, a new osteopathic hospital was constructed on Munson Avenue on Traverse City's east side. Traverse City Osteopathic Hospital later became part of Munson Hospital, and the building seen in this postcard was demolished in 1995 and replaced with Munson Community Health Center.

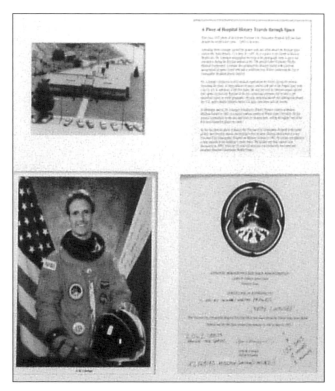

HOSPITAL PHOTO IN SPACE, 2004. This plaque hangs in the lobby of Munson Community Health Center (the former Osteopathic Hospital). The text on the upper right tells of how a c. 1955 photo (seen on the upper left) of the old Osteopathic Hospital circled the world 2,062 times. Astronaut Jerry Linenger took the photograph into space in 1997 and had it with him during his time on the Mir space station. This particular photograph had been placed in a time capsule during the construction of the Osteopathic Hospital in 1962, and it was removed in 1995. A Michigan native and current resident of the Grand Traverse area, Dr. Linenger completed a family practice rotation at Munson Hospital in 1981. A NASA certificate of authenticity is in the lower right.

Seven

OTHER PLACES
OF INTEREST

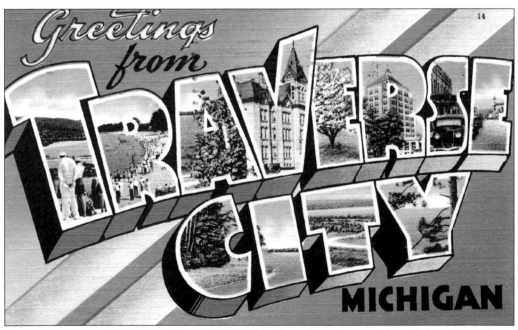

GREETINGS FROM TRAVERSE CITY, 1941. This "large-letter" postcard mailed in 1941 shows many of Traverse City's attractions and features. The Old Center of Traverse City State Hospital is found in the "V." This chapter will explore a few of the places in Traverse City with history related to the state hospital, and also some other institutions in Michigan and other states.

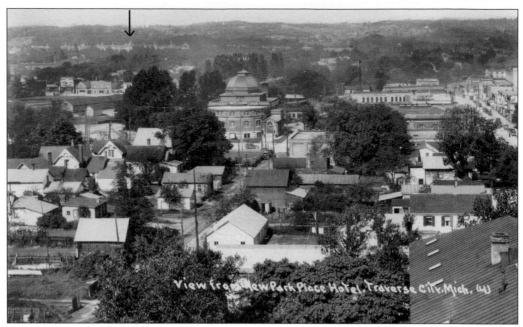

VIEW FROM THE PARK PLACE HOTEL. This postcard from the 1920s shows an aerial view of western Traverse City from the vantage point of the Park Place Hotel downtown. The white line in the upper left background represents the state hospital buildings. The black arrow points to Old Center. The Park Place Hotel is now much taller, but the trees have grown as well; in 2004, little can be seen of the state hospital buildings from the top of the Park Place.

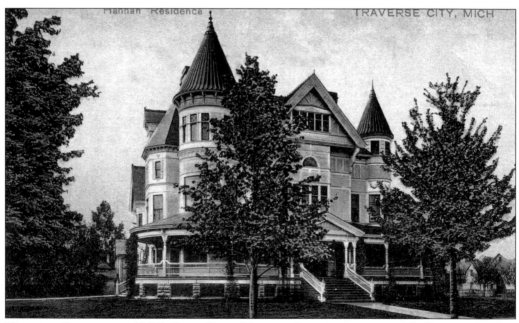

HANNAH RESIDENCE, 1907. Perry Hannah's magnificent mansion on 6th Street is another major architectural attraction in Traverse City. Designed by Grand Rapids architect W.G. Robinson, it was completed in 1893. Now a funeral home, the exterior looks today much as it did at the time of this 1907 postcard.

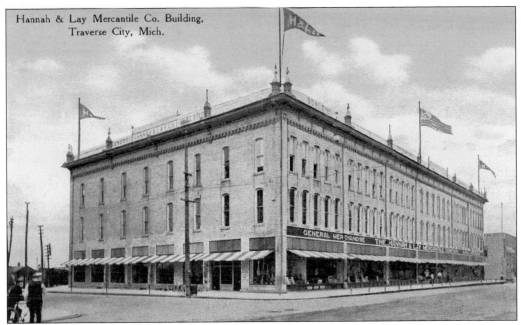

Hannah & Lay Mercantile Co. Building,
Traverse City, Mich.

HANNAH & LAY MERCANTILE, 1910. Perry Hannah's Hannah & Lay Mercantile in downtown Traverse City was built in 1883 with bricks from the Markham brickyards in Leelanau County. The same brickyard supplied bricks for Building 50 and many other state hospital buildings.

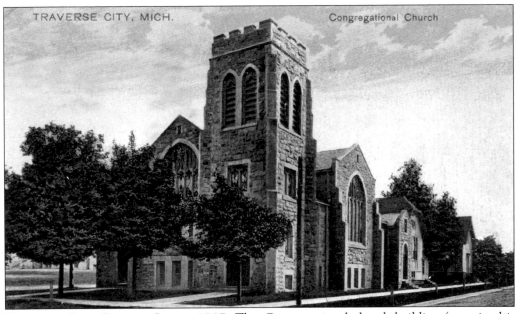

TRAVERSE CITY, MICH. Congregational Church

TRAVERSE CITY CHURCH LAND, 1907. This Congregational church building (seen in this 1907 postcard) was built on land originally donated by Perry Hannah. Just behind the church building, on the right, is the synagogue of Congregation Beth-El, also located on land donated by Perry Hannah. It was opened in 1885 (the same year as Northern Michigan Asylum) and is now the oldest operating synagogue in the state of Michigan. First Congregational Church left this church building in 1960.

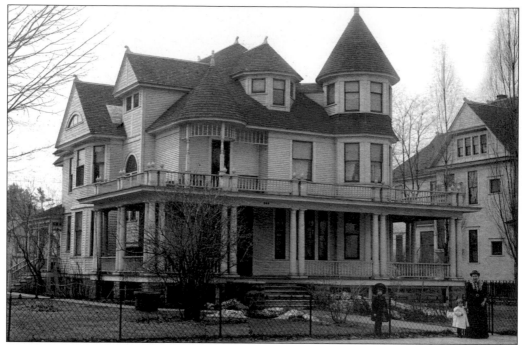

CUYLER GERMAIN HOME, 1911. 333 Sixth Street was the home of Cuyler Germaine, a long-time Hannah Lay employee. His son, William "Wild Bill" Germaine, married into the Hulls, another prominent family and owners of the Oval Wood Dish Factory. William, one of the more colorful characters in Traverse City's early history, ended up at Northern Michigan Asylum. This postcard from 1911 is from Anna Kratochvil Germaine to Mrs. Frank Kratochvil and family.

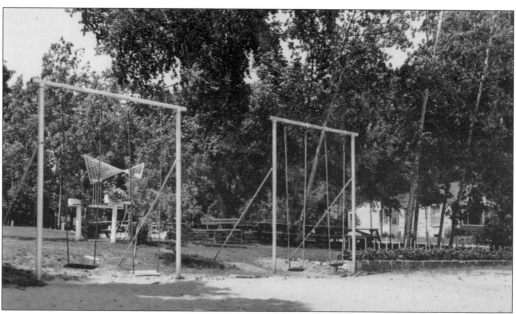

STATE HOSPITAL PARK IN LEELANAU COUNTY. For many years, the state hospital owned a park on Grand Traverse Bay in Bingham Township, Leelanau County. It is now a township park.

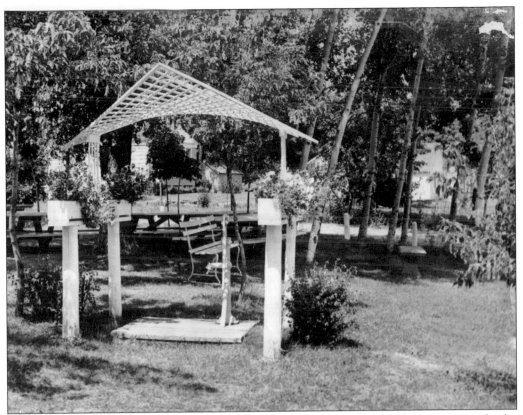

PICNIC GROUNDS. This photograph from the time of the hospital's operation shows the cover for the pump at the state hospital picnic grounds (looking north by west). (Courtesy of Julius Petertyl.)

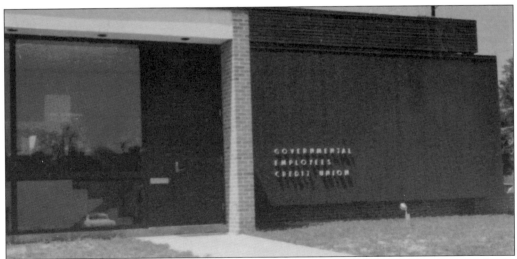

GOVERNMENT EMPLOYEES' CREDIT UNION. Traverse City Governmental Employees Credit Union was founded in 1954 to serve state hospital and other government employees. It started out in the basement of Old Center. The Beaumont Street branch building, shown in this 1967 photo, was constructed between 1965 and 1967. This financial institution is now known as Members Credit Union. (Courtesy of Members Credit Union.)

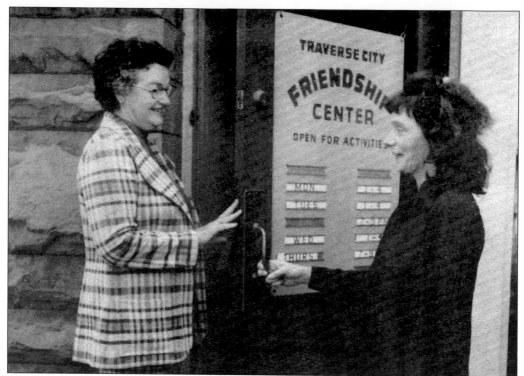

FRIENDSHIP CENTER ENTRANCE, 1973. The Traverse City Friendship Center opened on September 17, 1973, to provide a "drop-in center for social activities for released state hospitals patients now living in the communities, or for other socio-emotionally handicapped persons." It was located on the second floor of the City Opera House in downtown Traverse City. In this photo from a special edition of *The Observer*, a volunteer welcomes a member.

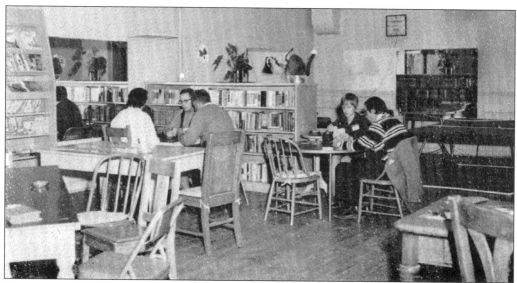

FRIENDSHIP CENTER SOCIAL ROOM, 1973. Friendship Center members participate in activities in the furnished social room of the Friendship Center. This space had previously been a dance studio, and all furniture, books, and records were donated to the effort.

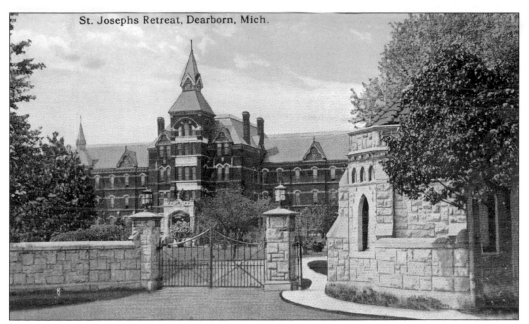

POSTCARD VIEW OF ST. JOSEPH'S RETREAT, 1919. St. Joseph's Retreat in Dearborn was Michigan's first private psychiatric hospital. It was started by the Daughters of Charity of St. Vincent de Paul. The 1885 building shown here was influenced by the Kirkbride plan. St. Joseph's was demolished in 1963.

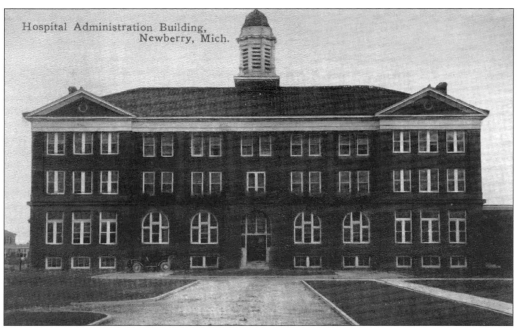

POSTCARD OF NEWBERRY STATE HOSPITAL, 1910. Newberry State Hospital opened in the mid-1890s in the eastern Upper Peninsula of Michigan. This one stayed open for a few years longer than Traverse City State Hospital, and closed in 1992. Much of it has now been converted into a state correctional facility. Dr. Earle Campbell, who served as superintendent in Traverse City from 1924 to 1926, served at the Newberry hospital before and after this time.

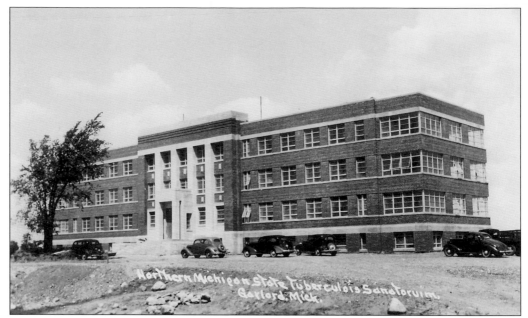

POSTCARD OF GAYLORD SANATORIUM, PRIOR TO 1942. The tuberculosis sanatorium in Gaylord (northeast of Traverse City) was built in 1937. In the 1960s it became the Gaylord State Home, a residential and training institution for people with developmental disabilities. Today it is known as J. Richard Yuill Alpine Center, and houses a variety of government offices.

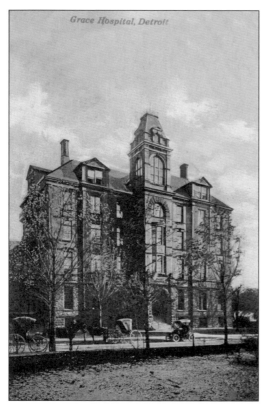

POSTCARD VIEW OF GRACE HOSPITAL, 1913. Grace Hospital in Detroit, Michigan, is seen in this 1913 postcard view. This medical hospital was designed by Gordon W. Lloyd, the architect who designed Building 50. The building has long since been demolished, but Grace Hospital survives (along with Children's Hospital, Harper Hospital, and others) in new buildings in a consolidated complex known as Detroit Medical Center.

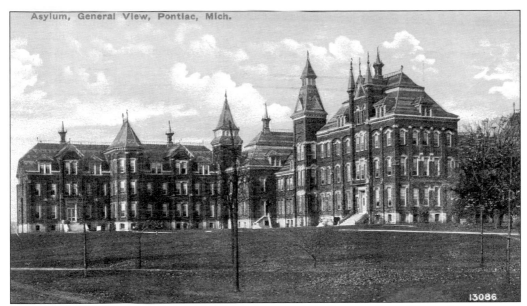

13086

POSTCARD VIEW OF PONTIAC STATE HOSPITAL, 1912. Pontiac State Hospital was known in its last years as Clinton Valley Center. It closed in 1997. It was located to the east of the Summit Mall area in Pontiac, Michigan. Despite a preservation fight and offers from developers, its historic Kirkbride-plan building (only a part of which is seen here) was demolished in 2000, along with cottages and other buildings.

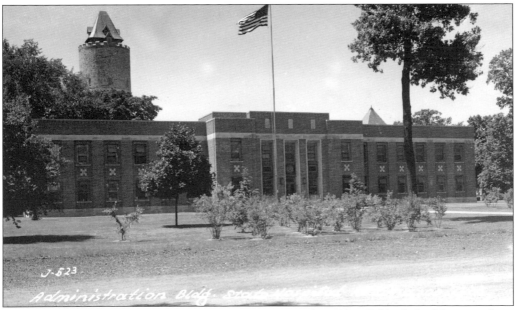

J-523

Administration Bldg. State Hospital

POSTCARD VIEW OF KALAMAZOO STATE HOSPITAL, 1950s. The Kirkbride buildings are long gone, but the distinctive water tower remains at what is now known as Kalamazoo Regional Psychiatric Hospital. The first of Michigan's large asylums is now the only one still in operation as a mental health care facility.

95

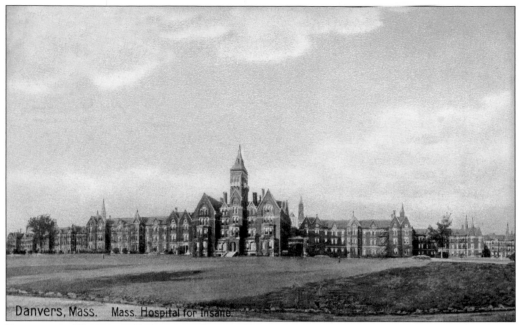

POSTCARD VIEW OF DANVERS STATE HOSPITAL, 1910S. Danvers State Hospital in Massachusetts first opened in 1878. It closed in 1992, and much (if not all) of the distinctive Kirkbride-plan main building faces demolition at this time.

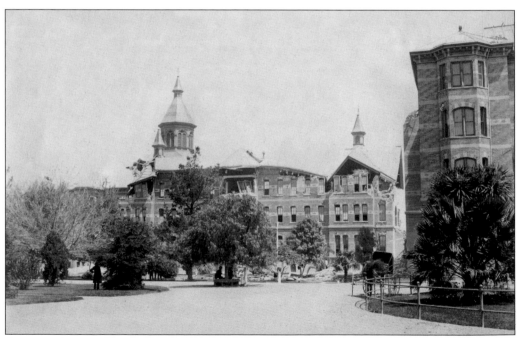

AGNEWS ASYLUM EARTHQUAKE DAMAGE, 1906. Agnews State Hospital, near San Francisco, was established in 1885 (the same year as Northern Michigan Asylum and other institutions). It was badly damaged during the earthquake of April 18, 1906. Some of the building has been renovated, and houses Sun Microsystems.

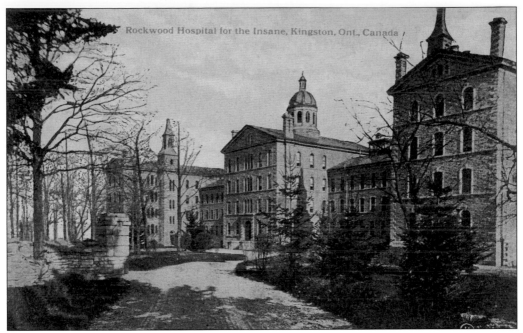

ROCKWOOD HOSPITAL, C. 1910S. While a large number of Kirkbride-plan psychiatric hospitals were built in the United States, several were built elsewhere, as well, including several in Canada and one in Sydney, Australia. This postcard view shows one in Ontario, Canada.

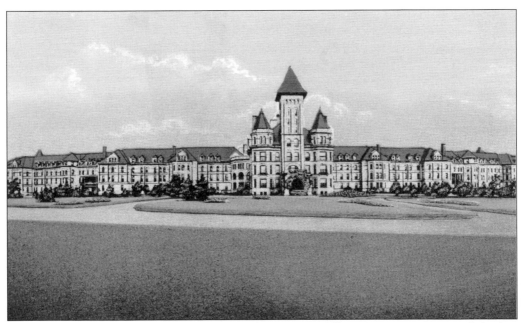

FERGUS FALLS STATE HOSPITAL. This building at Fergus Falls, Minnesota, was one of the last Kirkbride buildings constructed. It was designed by architect Warren B. Dunnell. Construction started in 1888, and the last part (the center section) was completed in 1906. It is the only one of Minnesota's Kirkbride buildings still standing, and it remains in excellent and complete condition.

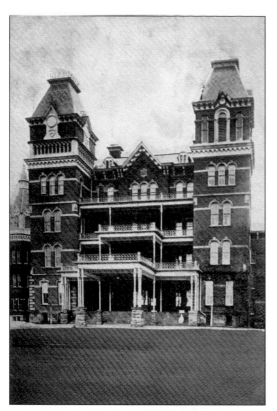

ATHENS STATE HOSPITAL, 1909. Athens State Hospital was opened in southeast Ohio in 1874. This postcard view from 1909 shows the center section of the Kirkbride building, which was designed by the architect Levi T. Scofield. The buildings of the former state hospital are now part of Ohio University, and this center section is now the Kennedy Museum of Art. Also in Ohio, the Kirkbride-plan building at the former Dayton State Hospital has been transformed into senior housing.

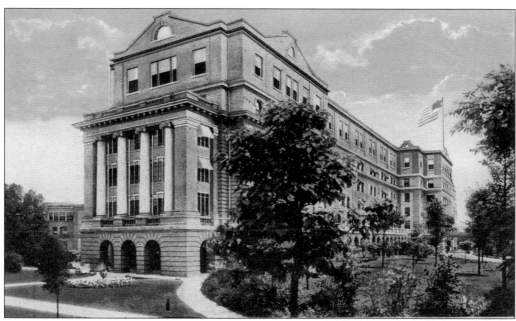

BATTLE CREEK SANITARIUM, 1923. This postcard view from 1923 shows the Kellogg Sanitarium in Battle Creek, Michigan. This place, actually a health spa, was featured in the 1994 film *The Road to Wellville*. The buildings of Traverse City Hospital were considered for filming, but were ultimately not used. The former sanitarium is now a federal document repository.

Eight

Traverse City
State Hospital
1885–1989

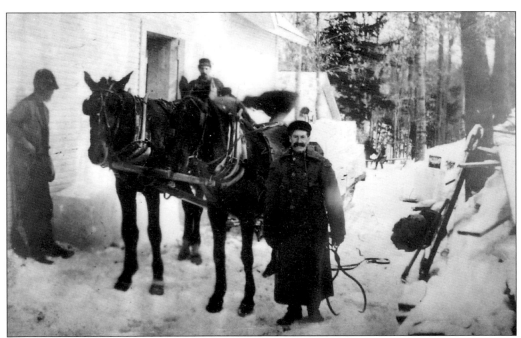

ICE WORK CREW. This photo from the early years of the asylum shows men working with ice on what is now Yellow Drive in front of the root cellar buildings to the west of the service buildings. This chapter covers people and events from the institution's 104-year history, including aerial photos and maps from various years. (Courtesy of the State Archives of Michigan.)

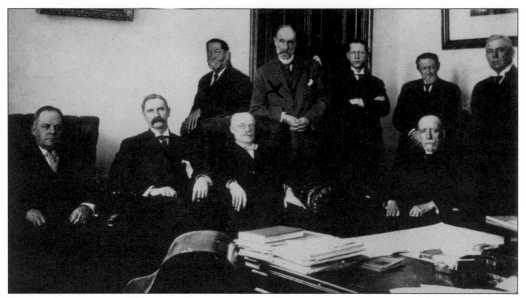

POSTCARD OF STATE HOSPITAL BOARD, 1909. Dr. Munson (center) poses for a photograph with the eight other men who made up the state hospital board in 1909. This photo was probably taken in the trustees' parlor in Old Center. (Courtesy of the Grand Traverse Pioneer and Historical Society.)

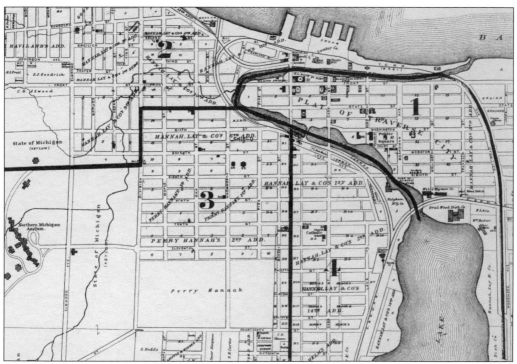

WESTERN SIDE OF TRAVERSE CITY, 1895. This map from 1895 shows Traverse City during a period of great growth. The asylum, seen on the left edge, has already added several of the cottage buildings. This map can be compared to the one on Page 9, which shows the same area in 1851. (Courtesy of the Grand Traverse Pioneer and Historical Society.)

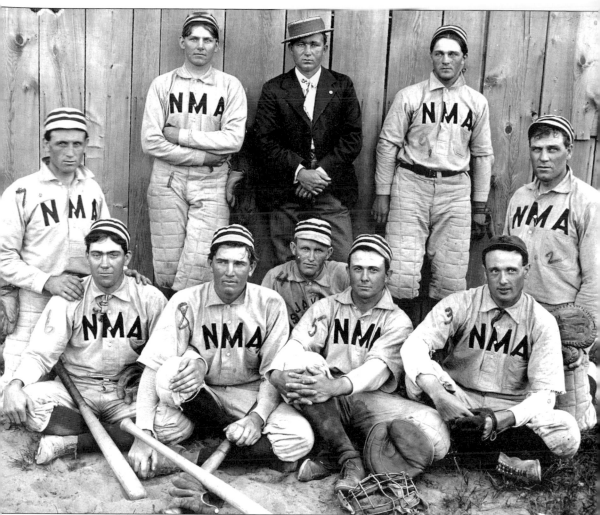

ASYLUM BASEBALL TEAM, 1900. This photograph from 1900 shows the Northern Michigan Asylum baseball team. The asylum also had a football team that at least once played against the local high school team. Names pencilled in on the back correspond to numbers seen in the photo. The names of these men are as follows: (front row, kneeling or sitting) 7. Al Ross, 6. Husky __ith, 8. Al Teuvy (?), 4. Ted Thirlby, 5. Otto Kistler ?, 3. Harry Baker, 2. Dave Cox; (back row) 1. Asa ? Cox, unnamed man in dark jacket, 9.

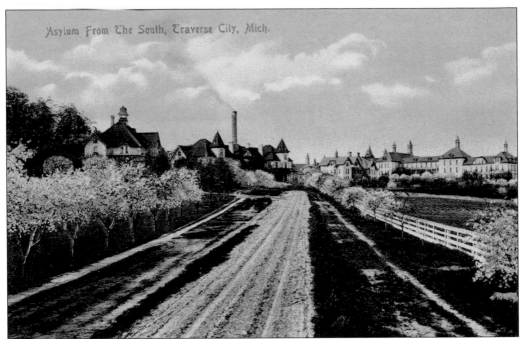

LOOKING NORTH ON SILVER DRIVE, 1900s. This Orson W. Peck postcard, *c.* 1906, looks north down Silver Drive. Building 40 is to the left of the road, and Building 28 is further to the left. Building 50 is to the right of the road, starting with Hall 20, and ending with the section now known as Southview at the far right edge of the photo. At this time, Southview was only two stories tall.

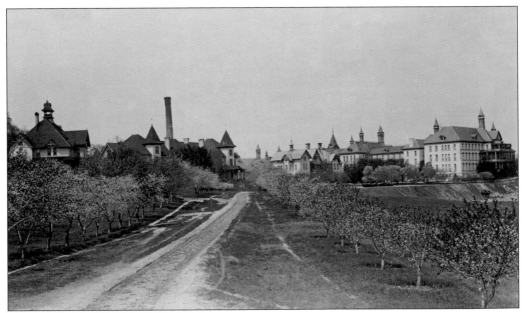

LOOKING NORTH ON SILVER DRIVE, 1910s. This postcard shows the same view several years later. The south end of Building 50 (seen on the far right) is by this time three stories tall due to a 1908 addition.

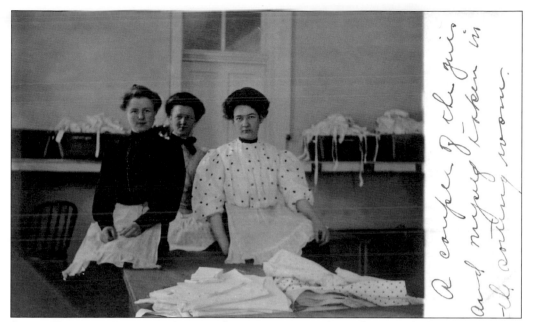

STATE HOSPITAL LAUNDRY ROOM. Three women pose for a photograph the laundry room in this postcard printed between 1904 and 1918. One of the women depicted wrote on the back: "I am well and happy. Work every day and go to church on Sunday. It is a very, very beautiful day today."

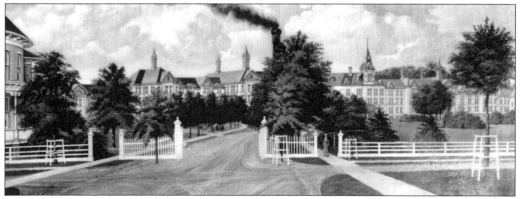

PAINTING BY ORRIE EDWIN CROWLEY. The painting shown above was painted Orrie Edwin Crowley (1865–1913). Originally a native of Iowa, Crowley made a living selling paintings after he moved to Isabella County, Michigan. He became a Traverse City State Hospital patient in 1906, after a mental breakdown. The actual painting measures 37.5 by 105 centimeters.

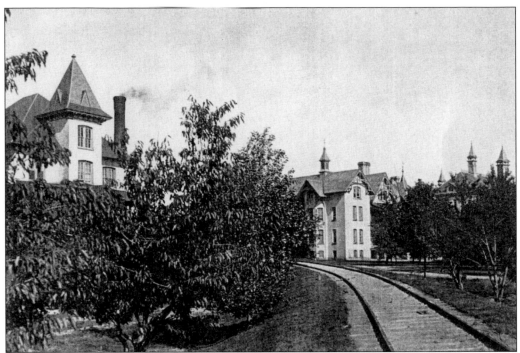

State Hospital Railroad. The hospital's railroad was constructed *c.* 1915 at a cost of $32,000, and in the first year of use saw 400 cars of freight delivered. The spur seen here, going between Cottage 40 and Hall 20 of Building 50, has been removed, but a small section of track remains embedded in one of the streets. (Courtesy of the State Archives of Michigan.)

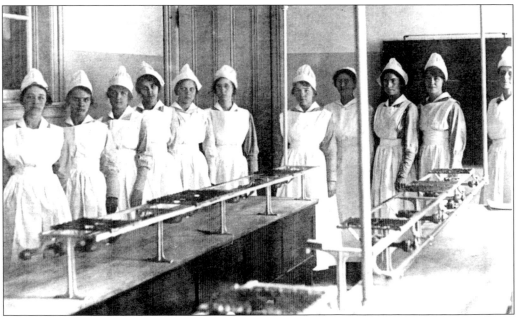

Diet Kitchen, 1918. This photo from 1918 shows the diet kitchen. It was utilized in the student nurse training program. (Courtesy of the Grand Traverse Commons Redevelopment Corporation.)

THE HERMIT. The man known to many as "Rock the Hermit" was born in Poland in 1846. His actual name was Roch Tybushewsky. According to one account, he accidentally killed a student when he was a teacher in Alpena, Michigan. He imposed the hermit lifestyle upon himself as a penance. He lived in Leelanau County, north of Suttons Bay along M-22, in a dugout. Even though he was a hermit, he ended up posing for a variety of photographs which were made into postcards in the first part of the 20th century. He was admitted to Traverse City State Hospital in 1919. He died there in 1931 at the age of 84. This particular postcard dates from between 1904 and 1918.

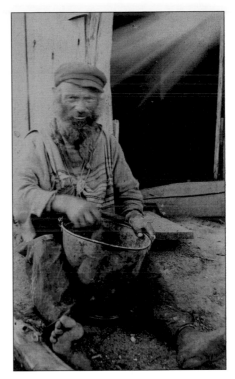

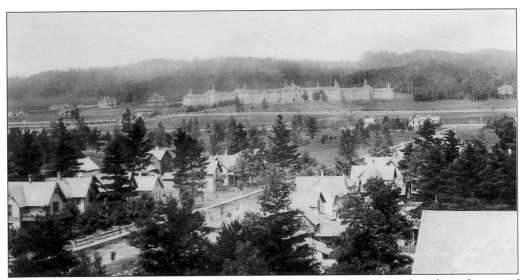

VIEW FROM OLD HIGH SCHOOL. This view of the asylum grounds was taken from the top of the Traverse City High School building. The site of the old high school is currently occupied by Central Elementary. The residences of the south side of 8th Street are in the left bottom corner. In the distance, the asylum buildings start with the "Special Barns" on the left (south) and end with Cottage 25 on the right (north). (Courtesy of the State Archives of Michigan.)

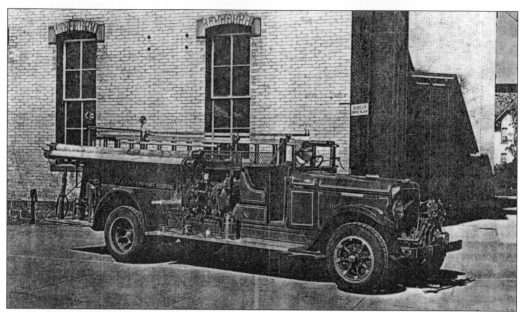

"OLD RED" FIRE ENGINE. The first fire engine was named "Old Red." The name "Traverse City State Hospital" can be seen above the rear right wheel of the truck. A state hospital publication in 1973 stated, "The danger of fire, from the very beginning to the present day, stands first in the list of concerns for patients' safety." (Courtesy of the State Archives of Michigan.)

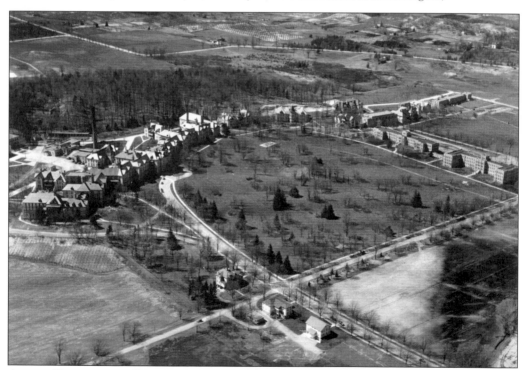

AERIAL PHOTO FROM SOUTHEAST, 1930. This photo was taken from the southeast looking northwest. Buildings 33 and 35 (on the right) had just been completed at this time. (Courtesy of the State Archives of Michigan.)

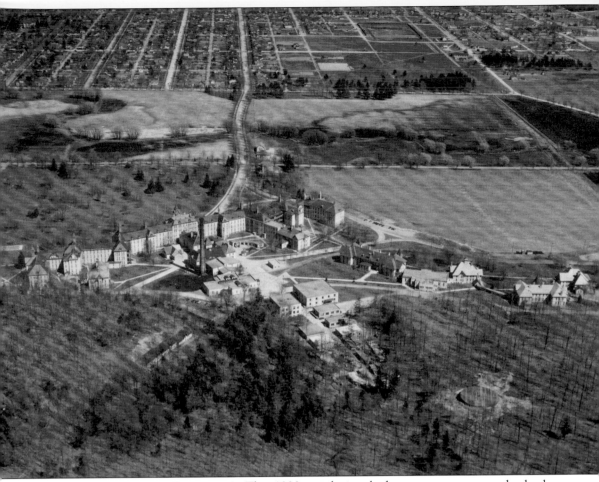

AERIAL PHOTO FROM WEST, 1930. This 1930 aerial view looks west to east, over the back of Building 50, with the Traverse City neighborhood north and south of 11th Street in the far background. A large number of service buildings can be seen here, including the ones closer to Building 50, which have since been demolished. (Courtesy of the State Archives of Michigan.)

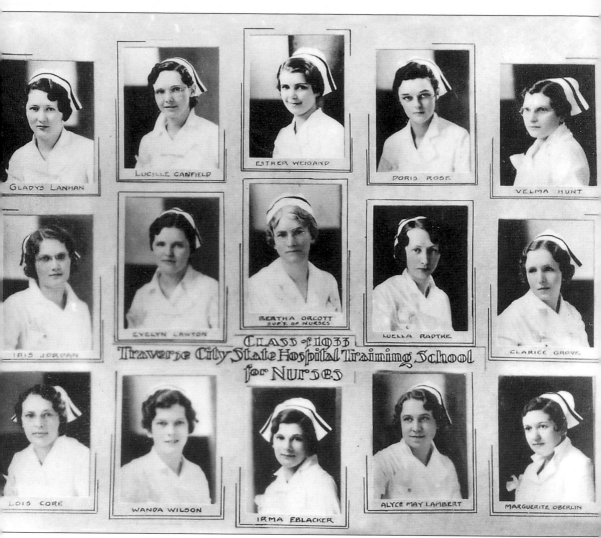

NURSE CLASS OF 1933. Dr. Munson saw a need for trained staff for the mental hospital, and as a result, a nursing school was instituted. In June of 1908, the first class of 24 students graduated. This class photo shows the nursing school class of 1933: (top row) Gladys Lanhan, Lucille Canfield, Esther Weigand, Doris Rose, and Velma Hunt; (second row) Iris Jordan, Evelyn Lawton, Bertha Orcott (superintendent of nurses), Luella Radtke, and Clarice Grove; (bottom row) Lois Core, Wanda Wilson, Irma Eblacker, Alyce May Lambert, and Marguerite Oberlin. (Courtesy of the State Archives of Michigan.)

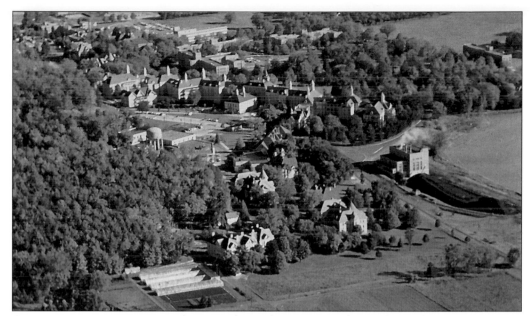

AERIAL VIEW FROM SOUTH. This view shows the main state hospital complex from the south during the early 1950s. At this time, the greenhouse complex (in the foreground) includes four greenhouses extending west. (Courtesy of the Grand Traverse Pioneer and Historical Society.)

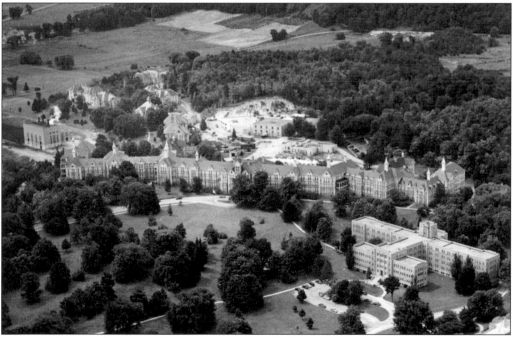

AERIAL VIEW, 1950S. This photograph shows how the main buildings of Traverse City State Hospital looked during the first half of the 1950s. The photo was taken after the construction of the new power plant, seen on the left edge of the photo, and before the construction of 37a. (Courtesy of Phil Balyeat.)

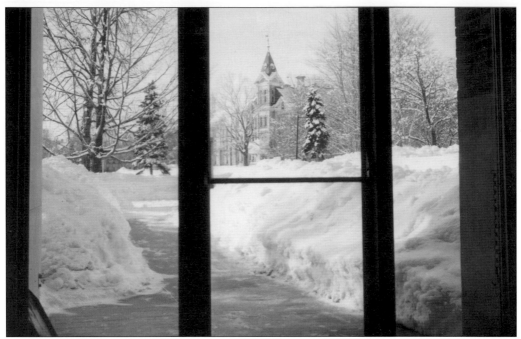

OLD CENTER SEEN FROM BUILDING 37, 1959. This photo from March of 1959 shows the old center of Building 50 from just inside one of the south entrances of Building 37 (the receiving hospital). Neither the view nor the vantage point remain, as the center of Building 50 was demolished in 1963, and Building 37 followed suit more than 30 years later. (Courtesy of the State Archives of Michigan.)

- **From Your Chaplains** -

Protestant - Chaplain George P. Dominick
Catholic - Father Edwin J. Frederick

For the time that you are here, we, your Chaplains, are interested in being of help to you. You have recently enter-ed a hospital, which is like every other hospital.

Nurses and attendants are here to help you. Doctors, Chaplains and other specialists will see you. These people are with you in your illness.

We extend to you our willingness to understand your deep longings within. Your feelings, values, loyalties, commitments and attitudes may be ones of emptiness, tiredness, or lost hopes. You have come to the Hospital with the feeling of needing help and we, with the cooperation of the Doctors, will give you every possible assistance.

Our experience makes us believe that you have a need to be understood and that being under-stood will help in your recovery.

A Chaplain will call upon you within the first few days after your admission. When you wish to see a Chaplain, ask a Nurse or Aide to notify us.

Sunday Church Services

Protestant Worship -- 9:30 A.M., Auditorium
Catholic Mass -- 7:30 A.M., Center Chapel

TRAVERSE CITY STATE HOSPITAL

CHURCH SERVICE BULLETIN. During the early 1960s, prior to the construction of All Faiths Chapel, mass was still held at the chapel behind Old Center and Protestant services were held in the auditorium in Building 39. Of the chaplains mentioned on the card, Chaplain Dominick would be replaced by Rev. Robert P. Bell in 1964, and "Father Fred" would remain on to serve the hospital and the community. (Courtesy of Julius Petertyl.)

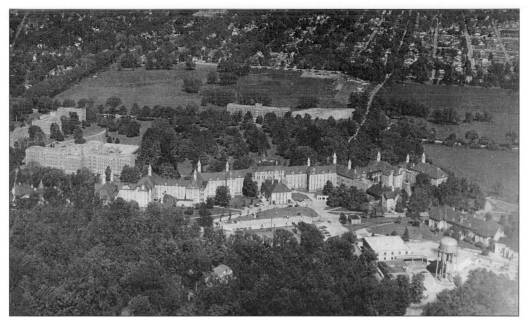

AERIAL VIEW, C. 1960. This image, taken from the west, shows Building 50 and the buildings behind it as they stood c. 1960, after the construction of 37a and before the demolition of Old Center.

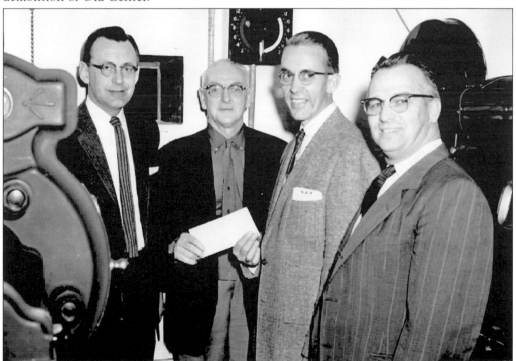

DR. SOMERNESS AND OTHERS. Standing with the state hospital movie theater equipment are Dr. M. Duane Somerness (State Hospital Superintendent from 1956 to 1972), Manager Jack Crawford, Warren Wardell, and Ohmer Curtiss (Director of Community Relations). (Courtesy of the Grand Traverse Pioneer and Historical Society.)

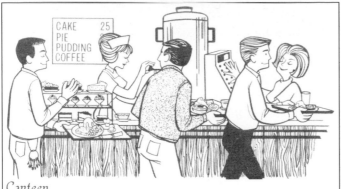

Canteen

The Hospital Employees Association operates a Canteen for patients and employees. The Canteen, which is located in Center Building, is a combination of sandwich shop and store. Many different types of sandwiches, plate lunches, beverages, baked goods and ice cream are available as well as a large variety of candy, tobacco, groceries and many other items. The Association also has vending machines for soft drinks and candy located in various parts of the hospital. The profits from the Canteen are split between the Patients Benefit Fund and the Association. The Canteen is open seven days per week.

STATE HOSPITAL CANTEEN. A section from the illustrated State Hospital Employees' Handbook tells about the canteen in the center section of Building 50. The chrome counter stools that were part of the canteen in 50a have been preserved as part of "Another Cuppa Joe" coffee shop.

"MENTAL HEALTH WEEK," 1966. This advertisement listed the events of Mental Health Week, which took place during the spring of 1966. Many of these flyers were printed up, and some turn up as backings for state hospital photographs. (Courtesy of Julius Petertyl.)

1966

VISIT TRAVERSE CITY STATE HOSPITAL

MAY 1 TO 7

Wednesday	May 4	Mental Health Career Day
Thursday	May 5	General Public and High School Tours
Friday	May 6	General Public and High School Tours
Friday	May 6	7:30 P.M. Evening Tours

Watch T.V. Programs

Channel 9 - April 19th and May 2nd - 1:00 P.M.
Channel 7 - May 6 - 7:00 P.M. (Limelight)

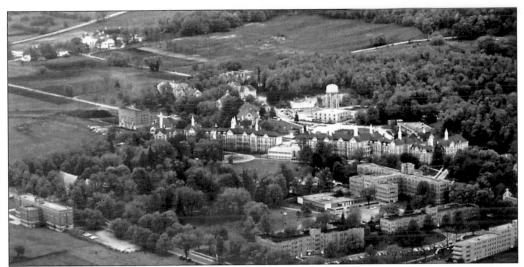

AERIAL VIEW FROM NORTHEAST, 1960s. This aerial view from the northeast shows almost all of the state hospital buildings as they stood at the end of the 1960s. The farm buildings, including the wooden cow barns, are in the upper left, and Building 41 is in the lower right. (Courtesy of the Grand Traverse Commons Redevelopment Corporation.)

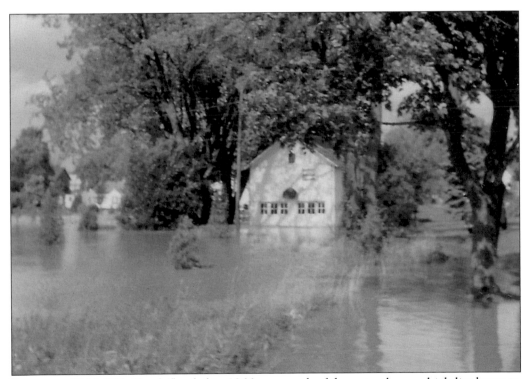

FLOOD OF 1966. Kids Creek flooded in 1966 over much of the natural area which lies between Division Street and the main buildings. The carriage house of the steward's residence stands in water in this photograph. (Courtesy of Julius Petertyl.)

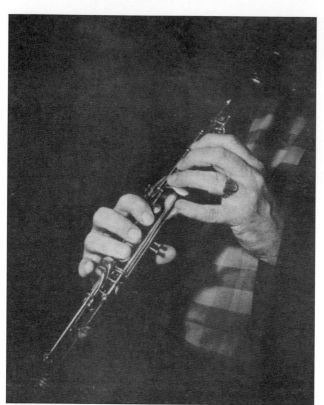

PLAYING A CLARINET, 1966.
This photograph is from "Hands as Therapeutic Tools," an exhibit of photographs that was exhibited in London, England, in 1966 at the Fourth International Congress of the World Federation of Occupational Therapists. The photographs were taken by Ohmer J. Curtiss. A booklet was printed by Gary L. Curtiss. The description for this photograph reads, "Producing a melody on a fine instrument may be an entirely new and thrilling experience to a tired and depressed business man." (Photograph by Ohmer Curtiss, courtesy of Heidi Johnson.)

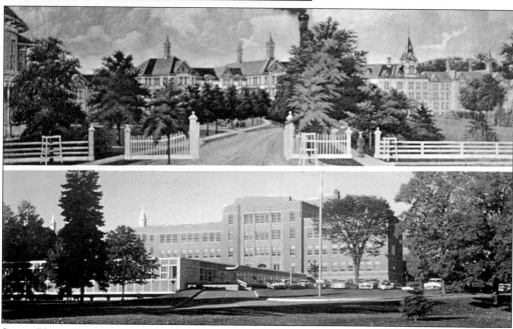

SPLIT-VIEW POSTCARD. This chrome-era postcard, likely from the early 1970s, is a split-view postcard. The upper view is from the Crowley painting (Page 103), and the lower view is from a photo of Building 37 (with the spires of Building 50 seen on the left). (Courtesy of George Beckett.)

114

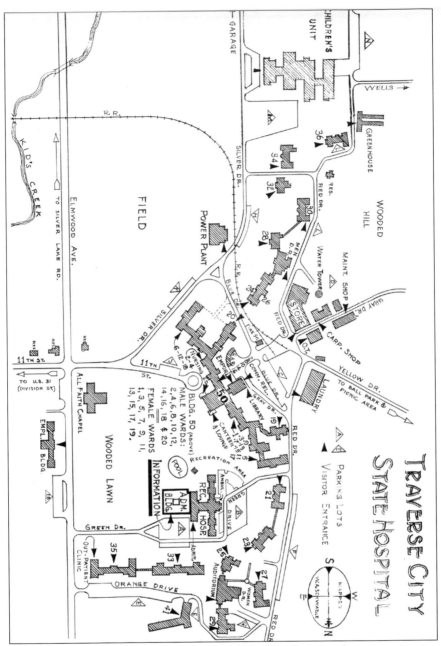

MAP FROM 1960s. This map from the Employees' Handbook shows the very active institution as of the end of the 1960s (after the construction of the new center and All Faiths Chapel).

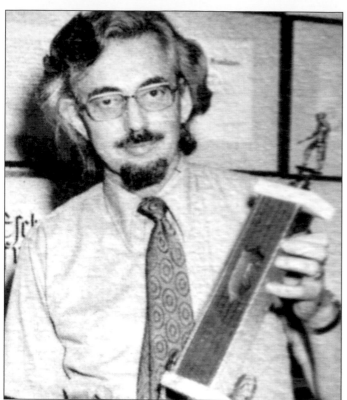

DR. PHILIP B. SMITH WITH TROPHY, 1973. The state hospital softball team took a second place prize at the end of the Traverse City Fastpitch Softball League's 1972 season. Superintendent Philip B. Smith is shown here with the trophy.

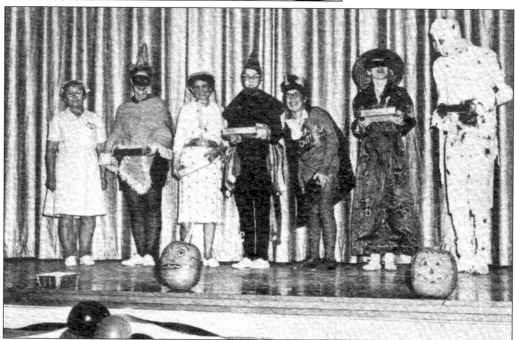

HALLOWEEN COSTUME PARADE, 1973. The costume parade from the Halloween program in 1973 is shown in a photo from *The Observer*. Winners received prizes from Mrs. Douglas, a Red Cross volunteer. The Halloween party was one of many parties and activities organized for patients.

THE LAST OBSERVER, 1973. A happy child opens a Christmas present on the cover of the December 4, 1973, issue of *The Observer*, which was Traverse City State Hospital's newsletter "for and by residents and employees." This was the final issue. An editorial inside reads, "As it is no longer considered relevant to the philosophy of our hospital, it was ordered to be discontinued." At the time, *The Observer* was published by the Activities Therapy Department, and had a circulation of 800.

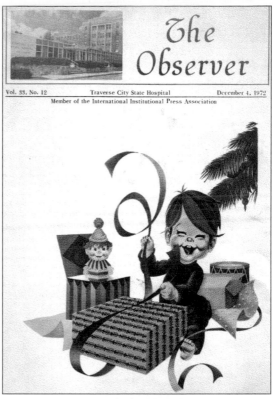

The
Observer

Vol. 33, No. 12   Traverse City State Hospital   December 4, 1972
Member of the International Institutional Press Association

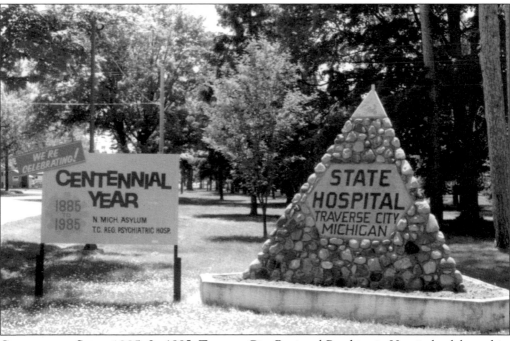

CENTENNIAL SIGN, 1985. In 1985, Traverse City Regional Psychiatric Hospital celebrated its centennial. A sign was placed at the southwest corner of 11th and Division next to the stone pyramid. (Courtesy of Paul Hansen.)

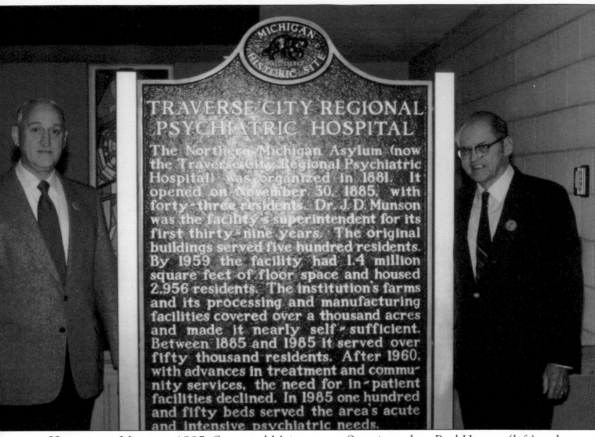

HISTORICAL MARKER, 1985. Structural Maintenance Superintendent Paul Hansen (left) and Grounds Department Superintendent Earle Steele (right) stand by the new historical marker plaque in 1985. It was temporarily inside the All Faiths Chapel, for the dedication ceremony. This plaque was placed near Building 37. It reads:

The Northern Michigan Asylum (now the Traverse City Regional Psychiatric Hospital) was organized in 1881. It opened on November 30, 1885, with forty three residents. Dr. J. D. Munson was the facility's superintendent for its first thirty-nine years. The original buildings served five hundred residents. By 1959 the facility had 1.4 million square feet of floor space and housed 2,956 residents. The institution's farms and its processing and manufacturing facilities covered over a thousand acres and made it nearly self-sufficient. Between 1885 and 1985 it served over fifty thousand residents. After 1960, with advances in treatment and community services, the need for in-patient facilities declined. In 1985 one hundred and fifty beds served the area's acute and intensive psychiatric needs.

(Courtesy of Paul Hansen.)

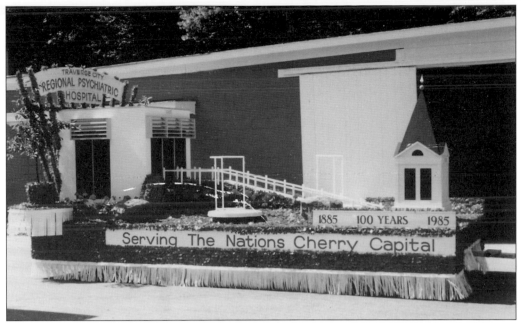

PARADE FLOAT, 1985. This parade float, seen parked in front of the machine shop building in the service building area, participated in the Cherry Royale Parade of the 1985 National Cherry Festival. (Courtesy of the Grand Traverse Pioneer and Historical Society.)

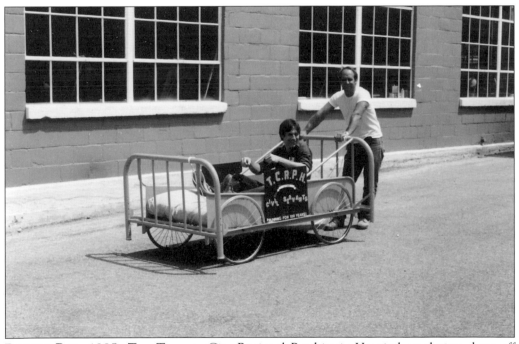

RACING BED, 1985. Two Traverse City Regional Psychiatric Hospital employees show off their racing bed in this snapshot from 1985. The bed races on Front Street have long been a part of Traverse City's National Cherry Festival. (Courtesy of the Grand Traverse Pioneer and Historical Society.)

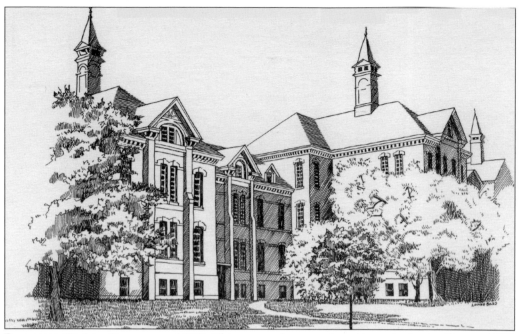

BUILDING 50 ART POSTCARD, 1987. This postcard was produced by artist Louise Bass in 1987. It depicts the southeast corner of Building 50. These are the sections which were renamed Southview and the Mercato as a part of the renovation of Building 50 into the Village at Grand Traverse Commons. (Courtesy of Louise Bass.)

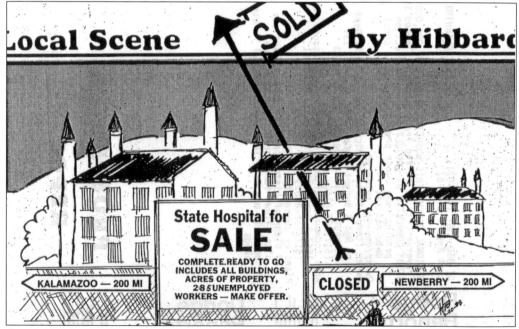

STATE HOSPITAL CLOSING CARTOON, 1988. This February 20, 1988, editorial cartoon is one of several concerning the state hospital that ran over the years in the *Traverse City Record Eagle*. The last patient left the hospital in August of 1989, and the hospital closed one month later. (Permission of Gene Hibbard and the *Traverse City Record Eagle*.)

Nine

REBIRTH

GRAND TRAVERSE COMMONS AND "THE VILLAGE"

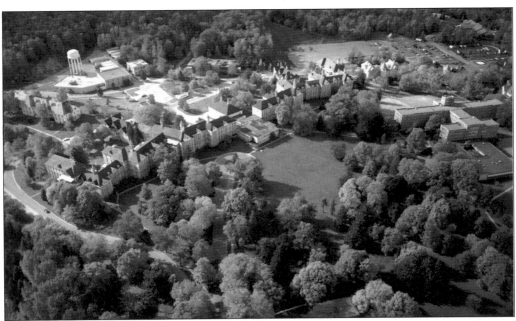

AERIAL PHOTO OF BUILDING 50, 1995. This aerial image from 1995 shows the Building 50 area just before major changes commenced with the demolition of Bulding 37 (right edge) and neighboring buildings. Starting in the mid-1990s and continuing through today, there has been significant development on the former Traverse City State Hospital grounds with new construction and renovation. (Courtesy of Jim Anderson Aerial Photography.)

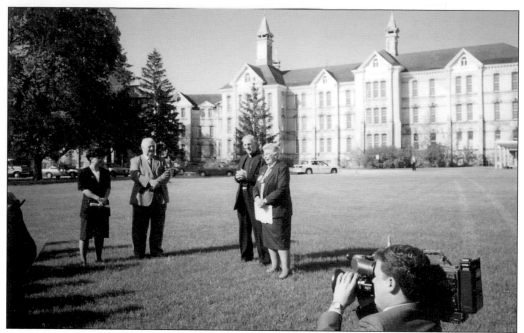

PROPERTY TRANSFERRED TO COMMUNITY, 1993. On May 17, 1993, Acting Governor Connie Binsfeld signed state legislation authorizing the transfer of the Traverse City State Hospital property to the GTCRC, the City of Traverse City, and Garfield Township. Pictured are, from left: State Representative Michelle McManus, State Senator George McManus, Father Erwin Frederick ("Father Fred"), and Lt. Governor Connie Binsfeld. (Courtesy of the Grand Traverse Commons Redevelopment Corporation.)

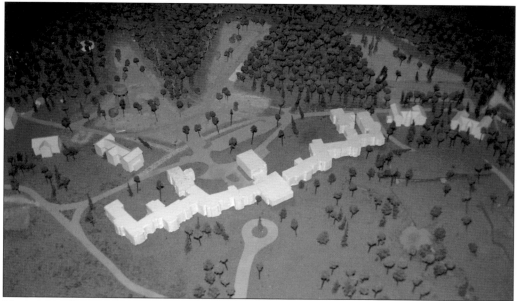

MODEL OF BUILDING 50. For its proposed development project in the mid-1990s, Kids Creek Development Co. utilized an elaborate scale model of the Commons property. This proposed development project was one of several to come and go prior to the Minervini Group purchase.

LAKE COUNTRY GAZETTE, 1996. In 1998, the Grand Traverse Commons Redevelopment Corporation (GTCRC) recommended demolition of Building 50, deciding that redevelopment was not feasible. The Committee to Preserve Building 50 (CTPB50) formed in the summer of that year to advocate for preservation. The fight for preservation was protracted, and was covered in newspapers such as the *Lake Country Gazette*, which covered this and other Commons controversies that had come before. A group of local architects and engineers also presented ideas that showed the feasibility of preserving the building. As a result of the groups' activities and advocacy, demolition was averted. It was not until 2001 that the GTCRC voted to convey Building 50 to the Minervini Group, which promised to preserve and redevelop it. In 2002, Building 50 received a new roof and redevelopment began in earnest. (Courtesy of Mark Stone.)

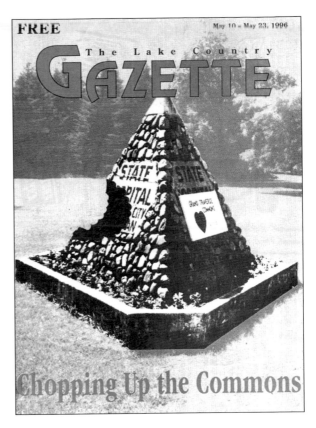

FREE   May 10 – May 23, 1996

The Lake Country

GAZETTE

Chopping Up the Commons

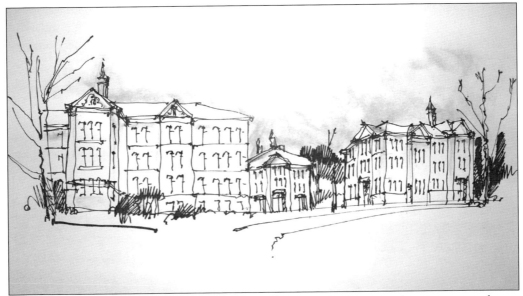

SKETCH OF SELECTIVE DEMOLITION. The efforts of a group of architects and engineers were key to publicizing the idea that Building 50 could be saved if it were renovated to mixed use, which would open up more opportunities for redevelopment. This sketch by architect Ken Richmond shows the center area of Building 50 opened up by the removal of 50a. (Courtesy of Ken Richmond.)

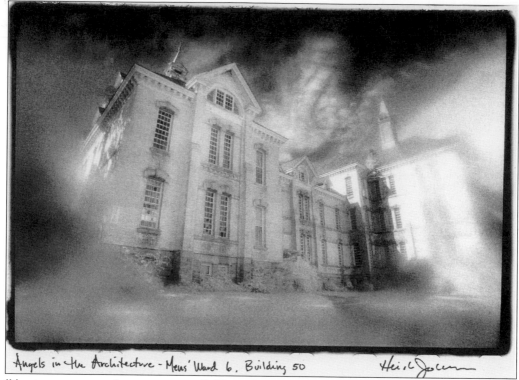

Angels in the Architecture - Mens' Ward 6, Building 50

"ANGELS IN THE ARCHITECTURE." This photograph by Heidi Johnson of the south end of Building 50 was the signature image for her "Angels in the Architecture" exhibition of photographs, and it was also used on the cover of her book by the same name. Her photography was very important in publicizing the beauty of the former state hospital complex at a time when its future was in doubt. (Photograph by Heidi Johnson.)

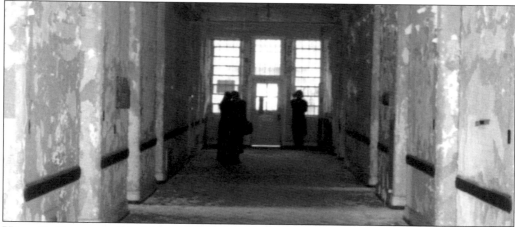

HALL 3, BUILDING 50, 2000. Hall 3 in the north wing of Building 50 looks typical of the unrestored halls of Building 50, In this photograph, three young women in black partake of one of the public tours offered in the late 1990s and early 2000s. The Committee to Preserve Building 50 promoted and helped with these tours in order to raise awareness of the building. The first-floor halls of Building 50 will house office and retail space (with the first opening in the spring of 2005).

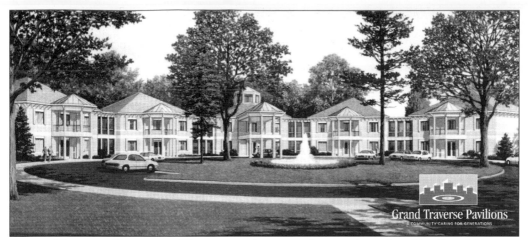

GRAND TRAVERSE PAVILIONS. This is one of a series of postcards produced by Grand Traverse Pavilions. The caption on the back reads, "Nestled on the park-like grounds of Traverse City's historic Grand Traverse Commons, Grand Traverse Pavilions offers a variety of clients a broad range of health care and residential options. The main structure consists of five rectangular pavilions emanating from a semi-circular inner pavilion. Included in the unique design concept are octagonal-shaped porches with weathered copper roofs, landscaped courtyards and terraces, and Italianate detailing." The Pavilions are located in the northeast corner of the Commons grounds on the former site of state hospital buildings 33 and 35. (Courtesy of Grand Traverse Pavilions.)

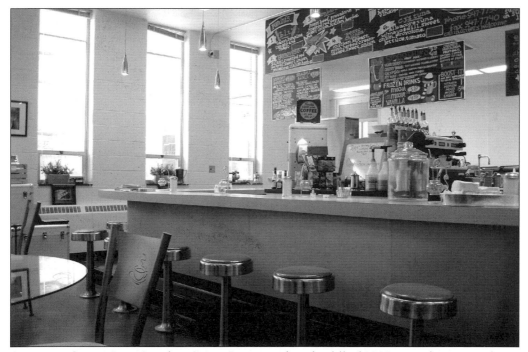

ANOTHER CUPPA JOE. Another Cuppa Joe opened in the fall of 2002, providing a significant amenity early in the Building 50 restoration project. The cafe is located in the former location of the canteen (page 112) and the old counter and chrome stools have been retained.

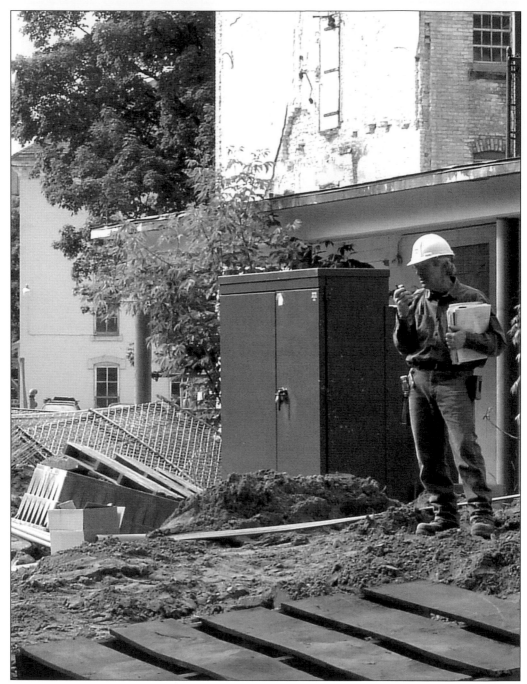

RAY MINERVINI, 2004. Ray Minervini, shown here at work in the southern rear courtyard of Building 50, leads the Minervini Group's renovation efforts. Their vision is to create a "walkable, mixed-use village that will feature a broad variety of residential and commercial opportunities." There will be hundreds of workers, hundreds of residents, and thousands of visitors each day. The Southview and Hall 20 sections are the first renovated sections to open (in 2005). "It's a matter of a building learning to become another sort of building," Minervini said an in interview with *Preservation* magazine.

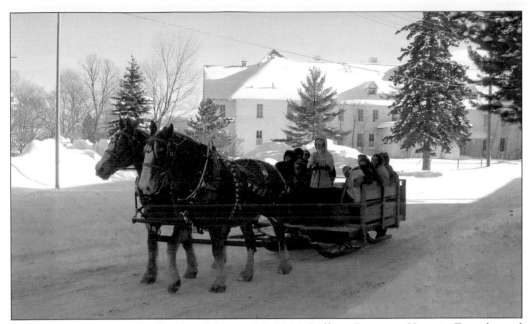

SLEIGH RIDES, 2004. On Sunday, February 23, 2004, Rolling Centuries Historic Farm hosted a sleigh-ride fundraiser. Here, a two-horse sleigh passes the back of Cottage 40.

PAINTING A SPIRE, 2004. During the fall of 2004, the spires on the southern half of Building 50 were painted, along with the spires on the chapel wing. Prior to this, they had been a dark rusty metallic grey for decades. In this photo, the Minervini Group contract workers apply primer. These spires are now white with "barn red" painted peaks and sandstone-color detailing. The Minervini Group's first task in 2001 had been to re-roof the building.

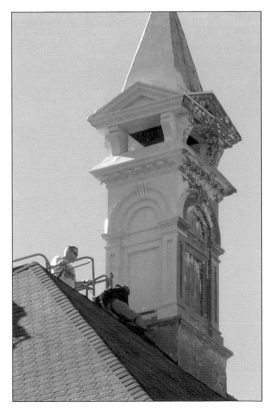

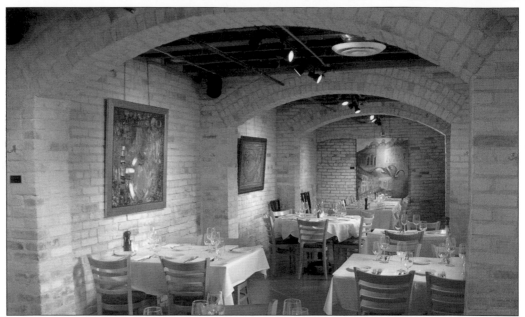

TRATTORIA STELLA, 2004. Trattoria Stella, which opened early in July of 2004, marked a turning point in the renovation of Building 50. The opening of this fine neighborhood-style Italian restaurant marked the first permanent occupation of the historic Kirkbride wings of Building 50 since it closed in the 1970s. Trattoria Stella is located in the garden (ground) level of Southview, the southernmost wing. (Photograph by Heidi Johnson.)

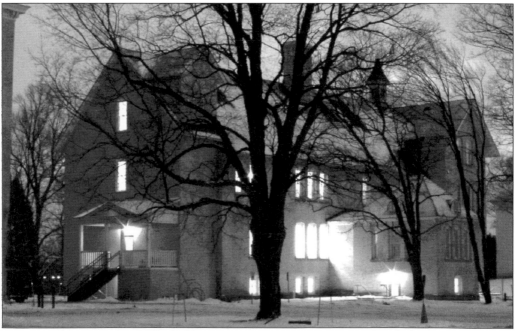

HALL 20 RENOVATED, 2005. Hall 20 is seen here at twilight just days before it re-opened in January 2005. Former Traverse City mayor and preservation advocate Margaret Dodd purchased the first residence to open up in the building. "I want to be where the action is," she said. "I love the concept of an indoor street 1/4 of a mile long with stores and services on both sides."